By Their Own Young Hand

of related interest:

Deliberate Self-Harm in Adolescence
Edited by Claudine Fox and Professor Keith Hawton
Child and Adolescent Mental Health Series
ISBN 1 84310 237 4

New Approaches to Preventing Suicide
A Manual for Practitioners
Edited by David Duffy and Tony Ryan
ISBN 1 84310 221 8

Suicide
The Tragedy of Hopelessness
David Aldridge
ISBN 1 85302 444 9

Hidden Self-Harm
Narratives from Psychotherapy
Maggie Turp
ISBN 1 85302 901 7

Promoting the Emotional Well Being of Children and Adolescents
and Preventing Their Mental Ill Health
A Handbook
Edited by Kedar Nath Dwivedi and Peter Brinley Harper
Foreword by Caroline Lindsey
ISBN 1 84310 153 X

A Multidisciplinary Handbook of Child and Adolescent Mental Health
for Front-line Professionals
Nisha Dogra, Andrew Parkin, Fiona Gale and Clay Frake
Foreword by Panos Vostanis
ISBN 1 85302 929 7

Understanding and Supporting Children with Emotional
and Behavioural Difficulties
Edited by Paul Cooper
ISBN 1 85302 666 2 pb
ISBN 1 85302 665 4 hb

Mental Health Services for Minority Ethnic Children and Adolescents
Edited by Mhemooda Malek and Carol Joughin
Foreword by Kedar Nath Dwivedi
ISBN 1 84310 236 6

Cannabis and Young People
Reviewing the Evidence
Richard Jenkins
ISBN 1 84310 398 2

By Their Own Young Hand

Deliberate Self-harm and
Suicidal Ideas in Adolescents

Keith Hawton
and Karen Rodham

with Emma Evans

Jessica Kingsley Publishers
London and Philadelphia

First published in 2006
by Jessica Kingsley Publishers
116 Pentonville Road
London N1 9JB, UK
and
400 Market Street, Suite 400
Philadelphia, PA 19106, USA

www.jkp.com

Copyright © Keith Hawton, Karen Rodham and Emma Evans 2006

The right of Keith Hawton, Karen Rodham and Emma Evans to be identified as authors
of this work has been asserted by them in accordance with the Copyright,
Designs and Patents Act 1988.

Library of Congress Cataloging in Publication Data
Hawton, Keith, 1942-
    By their own young hand : deliberate self-harm and suicidal ideas in adolescents / Keith Hawton and Karen Rodham,
with Emma Evans.
        p. cm.
    Includes bibliographical references and index.
    ISBN-13: 978-1-84310-230-4 (pbk. : alk. paper)
    ISBN-10: 1-84310-230-7 (pbk. : alk. paper) 1. Self-destructive behavior in adolescence. 2. Teenagers—Suicidal
behavior. 3. Youth—Suicidal behavior. I. Rodham, Karen, 1970- II. Evans, Emma, 1975- III. Title.
    RJ506.S39H39 2006
    616.85'8200835—dc22

                                    2006013532

British Library Cataloguing in Publication Data
A CIP catalogue record for this book is available from the British Library

ISBN-13: 978 1 84310 230 4
ISBN-10: 1 84310 230 7

Printed and bound in Great Britain by
Athenaeum Press, Gateshead, Tyne and Wear

Contents

Part 2 Prevention and Treatment of Deliberate Self-harm in Adolescents

List of Figures

List of Tables

Acknowledgements

Much of this book is based on a study we conducted in schools in England in order to examine the prevalence of deliberate self-harm and thoughts of self-harm in adolescents, and the factors associated with these. This study was made possible by a generous grant from the Community Fund. The study was carried out in conjunction with Samaritans. We acknowledge the support of Simon Armson, Jackie Wilkinson and Su Ray from that organisation. We also thank other members of the advisory group for the study, including the late Richard Harrington and Nicola Madge. The study was conducted in collaboration with the Child and Adolescent Self-harm in Europe (CASE) study. Some of the research methods used for the study were developed through this collaboration. The senior collaborators from the other centres involved in that study are Ella Arensman, Diego De Leo, Sandor Fekete, Kees van Heeringen, Erik Jan de Wilde and Mette Ystgard. Nicola Madge coordinated this group. We thank Philip Robson for help with the development of our measure of self-esteem, Louise Harriss for assistance with some of the analyses, Sue Simkin for helping us in the preparation of the book in several ways, Nicola Madge, Ann McPherson and Anne Stewart for their advice, Sarah Fortune for her comments on part of the manuscript and Tania Castro-Martinez for secretarial support. We also thank the Oxfordshire Adolescent Self-Harm Forum for permission to reproduce in adapted form its guideline for schools (Appendix III); Lippincott, Williams and Wilkins for granting us permission to reproduce in modified form Table 3.3, which was originally published in Rodham, K., Hawton, K. and Evans, E. (2004) 'Reasons for deliberate self-harm: comparison of self-poisoners and self-cutters in a community sample of adolescents.' *Journal of the American Academy of Child and Adolescent Psychiatry 43*, 82–87; the British Medical Journal for granting us permission to reproduce in modified form Table 4.1, which was originally published in Hawton, K., Rodham, K., Evans, E. and Weatherall, R. (2002) 'Deliberate self harm in adolescents: self report survey in schools in England.' *British Medical Journal 325*, 1207-1211; and Elsevier for granting us permission to reproduce in modified form Table 5.1 and Figures 5.1, 5.2, 5.3 and 5.4, which were originally published in Evans, E., Hawton, K. and Rodham, K. (2005) 'In what ways are adolescents who engage in self-harm or experience thoughts of self-harm different in terms of help-seeking, communication and coping strategies?' *Journal of Adolescence 28*, 573–587.

CHAPTER 1

Introduction and Overview

This book is about deliberate self-harm in adolescents. This is one of the most important social and healthcare problems for people at this stage of life. Deliberate self-harm includes any intentional act of self-injury or self-poisoning (overdose), irrespective of the apparent motivation or intention. The purposes of such acts include actual suicide attempts, a means of altering a distressing state of mind, a way of showing other people how bad a person is feeling, and an attempt to change the dynamics of an interpersonal relationship. This book provides an overview of the nature and extent of deliberate self-harm in adolescents, including causes and risk factors, and offers guidance on treatment and prevention. It is intended to be a practical and easily accessible resource.

In the UK, the extent of the problem measured in terms of hospital presentations of young people who have self-harmed has been recognised for a long time (Hawton and Goldacre, 1982; Hawton *et al.*, 1982b; Kreitman and Schreiber, 1979; Taylor and Stansfeld, 1984a,b). Based on figures from deliberate self-harm monitoring systems, somewhere between 20,000 and 30,000 adolescents present to hospital each year in the UK because of self-inflicted overdoses or injuries. Deliberate self-harm represents one of the most common reasons for hospital presentation of adolescents. After deliberate self-harm was first recognised as a significant problem in the UK during the 1960s and 1970s, rates rose so rapidly that dire predictions were being made about the future demands that this phenomenon, especially self-poisoning by girls, would place on hospital resources (Kreitman and Schreiber, 1979). In the event, the rates levelled off, with signs of a small decrease during the early1980s (Sellar *et al.*, 1990). However, there has been a further increase in rates in more recent years, particularly in girls (Hawton *et al.*, 2003c; O'Loughlin and Sherwood, 2005).

During the 1970s and 1980s, reports of increasing numbers of adolescents presenting to hospitals after deliberate self-harm also started to appear from other countries, especially in Europe (Choquet *et al.*, 1980), North America (Wexler *et al.*, 1978) and Australia (Mills *et al.*, 1974; Oliver *et al.*, 1971). Particularly high rates of deliberate self-harm in adolescents resulting in hospital presentation (equivalent to those in the UK) have been identified in France (Batt *et al.*, 2004), Ireland (Corcoran *et al.*, 2004; National Suicide Research Foundation, 2004), Belgium (Van Heeringen and De Volder, 2002) and Australia (Reith *et al.*, 2003).

Most acts of self-harm that result in a young person going to hospital involve overdoses rather than self-injuries (Hawton *et al.*, 2003a; Hultén *et al.*, 2001). In the UK, the drugs used most frequently in overdoses are analgesics, especially paracetamol (acetaminophen). In Oxford, in recent years approximately 60 per cent of overdoses by adolescents have involved paracetamol (Hawton *et al.*, 2003a,b). This certainly reflects ease of availability – paracetamol is present in most households and can be bought over the counter in pharmacies and a wide range of other outlets. Other drugs used relatively commonly in overdoses include psychotropic agents, especially antidepressants and tranquillisers. Self-injury most frequently involves self-cutting, especially of the arm, but other methods include jumping from a height, running into traffic, hanging and self-battery.

What is the significance of deliberate self-harm in adolescents? Clearly it represents considerable current distress. In addition, long-term follow-up of adolescents who have self-harmed indicates a very high rate of suicide attempts in young adulthood (Fergusson *et al.*, 2005b). Furthermore, deliberate self-harm is associated strongly with risk of future suicide, the risk of suicide in deliberate self-harm patients in general being elevated some 50–100 times that in the general population during the year after hospital presentation (Hawton and Fagg, 1988; Hawton *et al.*, 2003d). Follow-up studies of adolescent patients have demonstrated that such people also have a greatly elevated risk of suicide (Goldacre and Hawton, 1985; Otto, 1972; Sellar *et al.*, 1990). In a long-term follow-up study (mean follow-up period 11 years) of a very large sample of patients aged between 15 and 24 years, over half of all deaths were due to suicide or probable suicide (Hawton and Harriss, submitted). Studies of young people who have died by suicide also highlight the association between deliberate self-harm and suicide. For example, in an investigation of suicide in 174 young people aged between 15 and 24 years, 44.8 per cent were known to have a prior history of deliberate self-harm (Hawton *et al.*, 1999a) – the true figure could have been even higher. Similarly, in psychological autopsy studies (which include interviews with relatives) of young people who have died by suicide, between one-quarter and two-thirds have been found to have carried out previous non-fatal acts of deliberate self-harm (Brent *et al.*, 1993; Houston *et al.*, 2001; Marttunen *et al.*, 1993).

Attention to prevention of suicide in young people increased during the 1980s and 1990s, when it became apparent that suicide rates were rising in 15- to 24-year-olds, especially males, in several countries, including England and Wales (Hawton, 1992), Scotland and Northern Ireland (Cantor, 2000), New Zealand (Beautrais, 2003), Australia (Cantor, 2000), Scandinavian nations and the USA (Cantor, 2000). In more recent years several countries have witnessed a downturn in suicide rates, but rates remain higher than they were before the rise.

Young people have, therefore, been highlighted in national suicide-prevention strategies – indeed, increasing suicide rates in young people appear to have been a stimulus for development of such initiatives in several countries. Also, because of the extent of the problem of deliberate self-harm in young people, their specific needs have been emphasised in policy documents aimed at improving the hospital management of patients presenting with this problem (Royal College of Psychiatrists, 1998). For example, in the UK, the guide on self-harm produced by the National Institute for Clinical Excellence (2004) highlights the need for specialised services for adolescents. Guidelines for the management of adolescents following self-harm have been produced in other countries, such as the USA (American Academy of Child and Adolescent Psychiatry, 2001) and Australia and New Zealand (Australasian College for Emergency Medicine and the Royal Australian and New Zealand College of Psychiatrists, 2000).

For some years, it has been recognised that deliberate self-harm in adolescents is far more common than is reflected in hospital presentations. This evidence has come from school-based or community studies, such as in the USA, a large-scale biannual investigation, the Youth Risk Behavior Survey, which began in 1990. This showed, for example, that in 2003, 8.5 per cent of adolescents reported an act of attempted suicide in the preceding year. Only 2.9 per cent said that this had resulted in presentation to a doctor or nurse (Centers for Disease Control and Prevention, 2004). In a similar investigation in France, 9.2 per cent of adolescents reported having made a suicide attempt in their lifetime, only 21.9 per cent of episodes having resulted in hospital presentation (Pagès *et al.*, 2004). In a systematic review of studies of this kind worldwide, we found that the average frequency of self-reported self-harm acts by adolescents in different time periods were as follows: suicide attempts – 6.4 per cent in the previous year and 9.7 per cent during their lifetime; deliberate self-harm – 11.2 per cent in the previous 6 months and 13.2 per cent during their lifetime. In addition, an average of 19.3 per cent of adolescents reported having had suicidal thoughts in the previous year and 29.9 per cent in their lifetime (Evans *et al.*, 2005a).

Thus, it is clear that when studied at the community level, the incidence of deliberate self-harm is much more common than appears to be the case from hospital statistics. However, such information has been lacking for adolescents in the UK. Therefore, we decided to conduct a major survey of school pupils aimed at providing realistic information of this kind for England. We included a large number of schools, chosen to provide a reasonably representative sample of adolescents in terms of gender, ethnicity, socioeconomic characteristics, school type and school achievements. We adopted an anonymous self-report approach, since available evidence suggested that this would elicit the most accurate responses. We used a more thorough means of identifying deliberate self-harm episodes than had been the case in most other studies. We examined a wide range of potential factors that might contribute to self-harm, investigated help and treatment received after self-harm, and studied coping behaviours used by the adolescents. We focused the study primarily on 15- and 16-year-olds because at this age nearly all adolescents should be in education and, hence, available for study. We also reviewed all other studies that have been conducted regarding prevalence of self-harm behaviours and thoughts of such behaviours (Evans *et al.*, 2005b), plus those relating to associated risk factors (Evans *et al.*, 2004). This allowed us to put the findings of our schools study in a full international context.

All of this material has been used in the production of this book. The main reason we have written it is because we recognised the need for an up-to-date and easily accessible source of information on this topic. Thus, we have provided a detailed overview of the extent and nature of deliberate self-harm in adolescents, a thorough examination of risk factors for this behaviour, and detailed guidance on means of treatment and prevention. In particular, we wished to produce a very practical book that would assist readers in relation to their own needs and roles in this field. Although a major focus of the book is on deliberate self-harm in adolescents in the UK, the topic is considered fully in the international context, especially in relation to studies of a similar kind to our school-based study. Our systematic review of all the available studies worldwide has helped to ensure that our references to the international literature represent a balance of findings.

In the next chapter, we explain in more detail the reasons for our having conducted our schools study and describe how we carried out the investigation. This incorporates evidence about research methods that influenced our choice of approach.

In Chapter 3 we present the findings of the research concerning the extent of deliberate self-harm and thoughts of self-harm in the adolescents in our schools study. These results are compared with those from studies from other countries. We also examine the methods used for self-harm. We review the complexity of motivations that appeared to underlie the behaviour, contrasting the motives for overdose with those for self-injury, and also the motives chosen by boys compared with those chosen by girls. We address the question of whether the adolescents in our study presented to a general hospital (or other clinical services) after harming themselves, particularly in terms of factors that might have made hospital presentation more or less likely. The problem of repetition of deliberate self-harm is highlighted. Finally, we explore the impact of self-harm and suicide on family members and friends.

In Chapter 4, we address the important issue of what distinguishes adolescents who self-harm from other adolescents and what differentiates those with thoughts of self-harm from adolescents who do not have such thoughts. One of the most obvious differences is with regard to gender. We attempt to answer the question of why this might be. Other characteristics we consider are age and ethnic background. Subsequently, we examine a wide range of psychosocial and health risk factors, both from our schools study and from other studies in a range of countries. These risk factors include mental health and well-being, exposure to suicidal behaviour in others, such as peers and family members, and the media. We also examine the evidence for the influence of a range of other personal factors and experiences (e.g. sexual abuse, physical abuse, homosexual orientation), family characteristics and social factors.

Knowledge of help-seeking behaviours and coping strategies used by adolescents is crucial to understanding both the background to deliberate self-harm and the means of preventing the behaviour and providing effective help following deliberate self-harm. In Chapter 5, therefore, we explore help-seeking and coping in adolescents in general, and then go on to use the results of our schools study to compare adolescents who self-harm with other adolescents, including those with thoughts of self-harm that they have not acted on, and those reporting neither experience. We examine help-seeking in terms of whom adolescents feel able to turn to for advice and support, and both help-seeking and lack of it before and after acts of self-harm. We focus particularly on thoughts and attitudes that impede help-seeking.

In Part 2 of this book, we focus on the prevention of self-harm and assessment and treatment of those who have self-harmed. One extremely important aspect of prevention concerns what can be done in schools. This is the subject of Chapter 6. After examining the reasons for schools being a logical major focus for preventive efforts, we explore approaches in this setting in relation to three considerations. The first is what can be done to reduce the risk of self-harm, such as through educational initiatives aimed at changing attitudes, knowledge and coping skills. The second approach concerns identification and provision of help for adolescents identified as 'at-risk'. Finally, there is the question of what help can be provided in schools for those who have engaged in self-harm, and what can be done to limit the negative impact of self-harm and suicide on others. We include detailed guidelines for school staff, which have been produced through a consensus process involving school staff, clinicians and researchers.

Self-harm often results in contact with health services. These have a vital role to play in prevention of self-harm. In Chapter 7, we first consider the important role of general practitioners (GPs), including how general practice care can be made more attractive to adolescents and how GPs can detect adolescents who may be at risk. We then turn to the role of hospital services, especially emergency department personnel and psychiatric services. We provide detailed guidance on psychosocial assessment of adolescents who present to hospital following deliberate self-harm. We then consider options for treatment of adolescents after self-harm. This includes a range of poten-tial approaches, provided by personnel from various professional groups. Sources beyond statutory services need to be considered in the prevention and treatment of deliberate self-harm in young people. In Chapter 8, we begin by examining the role of self-help books and telephone helplines. We then turn to the Internet, which is attracting increasing attention in relation to its potential usefulness as a source of help for distressed youngsters and also as a potential source of danger, especially where young people might access sites about self-harm that do not necessarily have prevention of suicidal behaviours as a primary objective. Finally, we consider other types of media, especially literature, film, newspapers and music, and the roles they might have in encouraging suicidal behaviour as well as their potential usefulness in prevention.

In the final chapter, we summarise what we have covered in this book. We then turn to the future and look towards developments that could help tackle this important problem. These include initiatives at family, school, health service and other levels, such as the potential role of the media. In addition, we identify key research questions that need to be addressed.

As indicated earlier, we planned to write a very practical book that would be directly relevant to all concerned with deliberate self-harm in adolescents and one that would ultimately be a contribution to the prevention of this problem and to the provision of more effective care of those at risk or who have self-harmed. We are confident that after reading this book, the reader will know more about the phenomenon of deliberate self-harm. In addition, we hope that our more ambitious goals will also be realised.

Part 1

The Nature of Deliberate Self-harm in Adolescents

CHAPTER 2

Investigating Deliberate Self-harm in Adolescents

Introduction

This chapter focuses on the practical issues that we addressed when we were planning and implementing our study to determine how common deliberate self-harm and thoughts of self-harm are in adolescents in the general population, and the factors that are associated with these phenomena. In conducting such a study, it is essential that the design and methods are thought through carefully in order to ensure that the findings will provide an accurate picture of the problem. As the reader will see, given the focus of this study, this is not a straightforward task. We therefore had to consider several issues when designing the study.

We explain the decision-making process that we engaged in as we decided how best to collect the information from the adolescents. Having chosen to use a questionnaire, we describe how the questionnaire was developed and tested. Finally, we explore the issue of consent, before explaining in some detail the process of implementing the questionnaire study in the school context.

Clinical versus community-based studies

Garrison (1989) raised concerns about how far the information concerning the prevalence of deliberate self-harm that had been obtained by focusing on clinical samples could be applied to the general population. For example, Hawton and colleagues (1996) found that as many as 70 per cent of deliberate self-harm patients admitted to hospital in Oxford who had previously self-harmed reported episodes that had not received medical attention. In addition, Choquet and Ledoux (1994) found that although 6.5 per cent of their school-based sample in France had attempted suicide, only one in five of these had been hospitalised as a result of the attempt. The findings of these studies meant that hospital-based studies were potentially excluding a significant proportion of adolescents who had engaged in deliberate self-harm but had not reached the attention of clinical services. This highlighted the need for well-designed community-based research focusing on the prevalence of deliberate self-harm.

Until recently, no sizeable community studies of deliberate self-harm in adolescents in the UK have been carried out. With the exception of Meltzer and colleagues (2001), who conducted an interview-based study of over 4000 adolescents and their parents, the few other investigations that have been conducted in this field have been small. In a London survey of 529 girls aged between 15 and 20 years who were screened for evidence of depression, Monck and colleagues (1994) found that nearly 13 per cent had experienced suicidal ideas in the month beforehand. In a sample of 294 university students in Birmingham, 63 per cent of females and 45 per cent of males reported having had suicidal ideas, with actual acts of deliberate self-harm having occurred in 4 per cent and 1.5 per cent, respectively (Salmons and Harrington, 1984). In a subsequent survey of 318 Oxford University students, 35 per cent of females and 31 per cent of males reported having had thoughts of suicide. Self-harm by cutting or other means was reported by 10 per cent of females and 5 per cent of males (Sell and Robson, 1998). Thus, although prior to our study and that of Meltzer and colleagues in 2001 a few community studies had been conducted in the UK, they involved relatively small or atypical samples, which means that the relevance of the findings of these studies for young people in general was very uncertain (De Wilde, 2000; Yuen et al., 1996). Nevertheless, they did suggest that deliberate self-harm and suicidal ideation are likely to be common among adolescents in the UK, and highlighted the need to obtain accurate and representative figures for these phenomena.

We therefore decided to design a community-based study. In the light of the weaknesses of previous studies that we have identified above, we were particularly conscious of the need to ensure that we included as representative a sample of adolescents in order that the findings of our study could be extrapolated to adolescents in general in the UK.

The rationale for a school-based study

We decided that the best way to conduct a community-based study of deliberate self-harm in adolescents was to do so through surveying school pupils. By focusing on those in Year 11 (i.e. those aged between 15 and 16 years), we would be able to include as near as possible a total sample of adolescents, because this is the final year of compulsory education. It would be impossible to survey a representative sample of older adolescents, since many would have left school and moved on to a variety of other settings, including university, jobs, employment training schemes and so on.

Aims of the project

The specific aims and objectives of our proposed research were to:

- determine the prevalence of deliberate self-harm and thoughts of self-harm in a large representative sample of adolescents

- identify the factors associated with deliberate self-harm and thoughts of self-harm in adolescents

- explore the coping strategies used by adolescents in general, but especially those used by adolescents who engage in deliberate self-harm or who have thoughts of self-harm

- investigate whether adolescents who self-harm or who have thoughts of self-harm have contacted helping organisations or sought help from elsewhere and, if not, what impedes their doing so.

The ultimate aims were to provide a full picture of deliberate self-harm in adolescents and to identify means for prevention and better management of this problem.

Choosing an appropriate method of data collection

Having decided that we were going to conduct a school-based survey of adolescents, we needed to identify an appropriate method for carrying this out. Choosing the best method for collecting information of such a sensitive nature requires careful consideration. We therefore conducted a wide-ranging review of the existing literature to find out how other researchers had approached the issue of collecting information on deliberate self-harm (Evans *et al.*, 2004, 2005a). One thing we found from our review of the literature is that interviews have been used less often than self-report question-naires. Interviews are expensive in terms of both cost and time. This has implications for the scale of a research project. Interviews are also subject to what Lee (1993) called interviewer effects. In particular, two kinds of effect can influence the types of response obtained: the social characteristics of the interviewers themselves and the expectations that interviewers bring to the interview. Generally speaking, because the interview is a social interaction between people, it is subject to all of the influences that affect such inter-changes. Such influences are likely to be particularly important when investi-gating personal and sensitive information.

Other areas of potential bias lie in the characteristics of the interviewer compared with the interviewee. For example, respondents are thought to be more likely to provide honest and accurate information to interviewers who are, or appear to be, from a similar social group to themselves. A further problem with the interview method is that of the researcher versus therapist dilemma (Alty and Rodham, 1998). This is what can happen when the respondent finds the interview to be one of the few opportunities available to them to discuss at length their concerns, needs and feelings about the topic being researched. The interviewer may feel torn between a desire to follow the interview protocol closely and an equally strong urge to take a therapeutic stance towards the respondent. Finding interviewers who have the appropriate skills and characteristics may be problematic.

Furthermore, choosing to take an interview approach can have a signifi-cant effect on the findings. Our review of the literature suggests that respon-dents are likely to conceal very personal types of behaviour such as deliber-ate self-harm at interview. Although questions can be worded carefully to reduce this possibility, respondents are considered by some researchers to be more likely to provide what are termed socially desirable responses. This means that their answers may be shaped by their need to demonstrate to the interviewer that are normal and that they do not have characteristics that appear to be less than socially acceptable.

Research on issues such as interviewer bias, social desirability and per-ceived anonymity has supported the suggestion that the higher the per-ceived anonymity of responses, the less tendency there is towards socially desirable responding (e.g. Aquilano and Loscuito, 1990; Embree and White-head, 1993; Midanik, 1988). This notion is supported by the findings from our review of the international literature on studies of suicidal and deliberate self-harm phenomena in adolescents, which demonstrated that, in general, reported prevalence figures for these phenomena are higher in studies employing anonymous questionnaires compared with interview-based studies (Evans *et al.*, 2005a).

We concluded that an anonymous questionnaire rather than an interview would be the most appropriate tool for our study. The key advantage of the anonymous questionnaire lies in the fact that the anonymity provided to the respondents decreases the likelihood of them providing inaccurate but socially desirable answers. Anonymous questionnaires have been shown to be particularly suited to collecting information of a sensitive nature from adolescents. For example, Safer (1997b) and Shochet and O'Gorman (1995) suggested that it is entirely likely that a young person who would admit to suicidal thoughts or behaviours anonymously would be far less likely to do so if such an admission would lead to his or her identification. It has also been shown that when adolescents are the subject of research of a generally sensitive nature, anonymous self-report questionnaires are most appropriate (Saunders *et al.*, 1994).

Developing the questionnaire

While we were planning our project, we were also strengthening links with other European researchers who had an interest in deliberate self-harm. The idea was that a European collaboration could use the same questionnaire to conduct community surveys of adolescents in several countries. It was hoped that the collaboration would be useful in providing information about a range of aspects of the problem, including, for example, why the levels of deliberate self-harm appear to be particularly high among adolescents in the UK. We developed our questionnaire with colleagues from the European collaboration, supported by advice from other colleagues who had experience of school-based studies. The European collaboration became known as the Child and Adolescent Self-harm in Europe (CASE) Study. It was coordinated by the National Children's Bureau in London.

The questionnaire to be used in the study needed to be sufficiently broad and yet detailed enough to obtain reliable information about the occurrence of deliberate self-harm and thoughts of self-harm, about the main factors associated with suicidal behaviour in adolescents, and about help-seeking and coping strategies of adolescents (both in those who had self-harmed and in those who had not). In practical terms, the questionnaire needed to be of a length that would not be off-putting to adolescents and that would allow its comfortable completion in the space of a single school lesson of 40 minutes. The questionnaire we developed included 11 areas of information. These are described below.

Sociodemographic information

The adolescents were asked about their gender, age, ethnicity and household living arrangements. The issue of how to record a participant's ethnicity was debated at length. As the questionnaire was anonymous, we were keen that the pupils should not be asked to provide information that might lead them to having a sense that they could be identified. Clearly, this could have been the case if we obtained extremely detailed information on ethnicity. We therefore chose to use the following broad ethnic groups: 'Black', 'Asian', 'White' and 'Other'.

Health issues, smoking, and alcohol and drug use

The second area focused on healthy living. The aim was to introduce the questionnaire gently by exploring how healthy the adolescents felt their lifestyles were. Following a couple of questions about diet and exercise, there were more detailed questions about smoking, and alcohol and drug use. These were as follows:

- How many cigarettes do you smoke in a typical week?
  1. I never smoke
  2. I used to smoke, but I have given it up
  3. up to five cigarettes a week
  4. 6–20 cigarettes a week
  5. 21–50 cigarettes a week
  6. more than 50 cigarettes a week.

- How many alcoholic drinks do you have in a typical week? (One drink, for example, would be half a pint of beer, lager or cider, or a glass of wine, or one measure of spirits.)
  1. I never drink alcohol
  2. one drink
  3. 2–5 drinks
  4. 6–10 drinks

    5. 11–20 drinks

    6. more than 20 drinks.

- Please tick any of the following types of drug you have taken during the past month (i.e. 30 days) and the past year.

    1. hashish/marijuana/cannabis

    2. ecstasy

    3. heroin/opium/morphine

    4. speed/LSD/cocaine

    5. other drugs and substances (not including medication).

Stressful events and problems

The third area focused on a range of stressful life events that the adolescents may have experienced. If they had experienced the life event listed, they were asked to indicate whether this was in the past 12 months and/or more than a year ago. The life events we asked about were as follows:

- Have you had problems keeping up with schoolwork?

- Have you had difficulty in making or keeping friends?

- Have you had any serious arguments or fights with friends?

- Have you had any serious problems with a boyfriend or girlfriend?

- Have you been bullied at school?

- Have your parents separated or divorced?

- Have you had any serious arguments or fights with either or both of your parents?

- Have your parents had any serious arguments or fights?

- Have you or any member of your family had a serious illness or accident?

- Have any close friends had a serious illness or accident?

- Have you been seriously physically abused?

- Have you been in trouble with the police?

- Has anyone among your immediate family (mother, father, brother, sister) died?

- Has anyone close to you died?

- Has anyone among your family or friends committed suicide?

- Has anyone among your family attempted suicide or deliberately harmed themselves?

- Has anyone among your close friends attempted suicide or deliberately harmed themselves?

- Have you had worries about your sexual orientation (i.e. that you may be gay or bisexual)?

- Has anyone forced you (i.e. physically or verbally) to engage in sexual activities against your will?

- Has any other distressing event occurred involving you, your family or close friends?

Deliberate self-harm

The questionnaire then turned to the issue of deliberate self-harm. The adolescents were asked whether they had ever deliberately taken an overdose or tried to harm themselves in some way. If they answered 'No' to this question, they were directed to a later section of the questionnaire.

Those that reported having engaged in deliberate self-harm were asked whether this had happened on one occasion or more often. They were then asked several questions about the last time that they had carried out an act of deliberate self-harm. The adolescents were asked to describe in their own words what they had done to themselves. Previous studies have generally not attempted to do this, instead simply asking whether a participant has engaged in deliberate self-harm. We decided that asking the adolescents for a description was important because it would allow us to determine whether what they considered to be self-harm met predetermined criteria for deliberate self-harm. For example, we would be able to exclude cases from our analysis where participants had clearly misunderstood what the term 'deliberate self-harm' meant. Thus, in the example below, the participant gave a detailed explanation of what she did whenever she hurt herself. However, this is clearly not a case of deliberate self-harm and was excluded from the analysis:

Paracetamol for headache. Pain killers – if I had a sore throat or gum pain. TCP when I cut myself, for example, cut my finger with the knife by accident when I was cutting something.

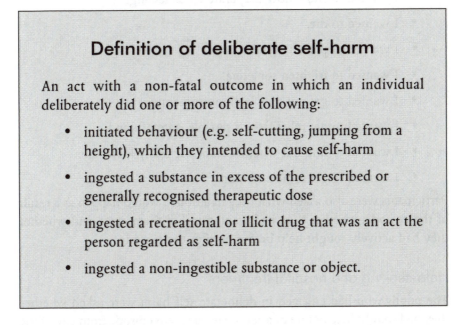

Definition of deliberate self-harm

An act with a non-fatal outcome in which an individual deliberately did one or more of the following:

- initiated behaviour (e.g. self-cutting, jumping from a height), which they intended to cause self-harm

- ingested a substance in excess of the prescribed or generally recognised therapeutic dose

- ingested a recreational or illicit drug that was an act the person regarded as self-harm

- ingested a non-ingestible substance or object.

The definition of self-harm we used in this study (see box above) was adapted from that used in a study focusing on episodes of deliberate self-harm in people of all ages that resulted in hospital presentation in centres throughout Europe (Platt *et al.*, 1992; Schmidtke *et al.*, 1996).

In collaboration with our colleagues from the CASE Study, we developed a manual to assist in deciding whether the descriptions of behaviour by the adolescents met our criteria. This is included in Appendix I.

Motives for deliberate self-harm

An important aspect of understanding the factors that lead to deliberate self-harm is an examination of the motives involved. Participants completing our questionnaire were asked to describe in their own words why they did what they did. They were also asked to choose from a list of eight motives or intentions those that they felt explained why they had carried out the act. The adolescents could choose more than one reason if more than one applied. The list was based on that used in studies by Bancroft and colleagues (1976, 1979). In these investigations, the motives were shown on separate cards. In other studies, as in our questionnaire, they have been presented as a list (Hjelmeland *et al.*, 2002), as follows:

- I wanted to show how desperate I was feeling.

- I wanted to die.

- I wanted to punish myself.

- I wanted to frighten someone.

- I wanted to get my own back on someone.

- I wanted to get relief from a terrible state of mind.

- I wanted to find out whether someone really loved me.

- I wanted to get some attention.

Participants were also asked what they had hoped would happen as a result of the episode, whether they had wanted to kill themselves, and whether they had actively sought help before or after the episode.

Help-seeking and hospital treatment

The pupils who had engaged in deliberate self-harm were asked whether they had sought help before or after the most recent episode from any of the following sources:

- someone in their family

- friend

- teacher

- GP (family doctor)

- social worker

- psychologist/psychiatrist

- telephone helpline

- drop-in/advice centre

- other source, e.g. Internet, book, magazine, other person.

We also asked the adolescents who had self-harmed whether they had been to hospital the last time they had done this, and whether they had ever gone to hospital as a result of a deliberate self-harm episode. This was an important question, because it enabled us to determine how many of our participants had not gone to hospital following their self-harm episodes and would, therefore, have been excluded from studies based entirely on hospital admissions to describe the prevalence of deliberate self-harm. It also allowed us to compare the patterns of self-harm (e.g. methods, motives) in those who reported presenting to hospital and those who did not.

Thoughts of self-harm

All of the adolescents were asked to answer questions about thoughts of self-harm. They were asked whether they had ever seriously *thought* about taking an overdose or harming themselves but not actually engaged in the act of deliberate self-harm. They were also asked whether they had sought help after experiencing thoughts of self-harm and about the sources of this help.

Coping strategies

A further part of the questionnaire focused on the coping strategies that the adolescents employed when they were worried or upset, asking them how often (never, sometimes, often) they did any of the following:

- talk to someone
- blame myself
- get angry
- stay in my room
- think about how I have dealt with similar situations
- have an alcoholic drink
- try not to think about what is worrying me
- try to sort things out.

The questionnaire then asked whom the adolescents felt they could talk to about things that really bothered them:

- father/stepfather
- mother/stepmother
- brother/sister

- another relative
- friend
- teacher
- somebody else.

Psychological characteristics

The next section of the questionnaire focused on the adolescents' current mood state. To assess mood, we used the Hospital Anxiety and Depression Scale (HADS). This is a reliable and user-friendly 14-item scale for measuring levels of depression and anxiety in non-psychiatric populations (Zigmond and Snaith, 1983), which has been validated for use with adolescents (White *et al.*, 1999).

We also incorporated a shortened eight-item version of Robson's (1989) Self Concept Scale to measure the adolescents' levels of self-esteem. This scale was developed in collaboration with Robson; it is included in Appendix IV. In addition, we assessed how impulsive the adolescents felt they were. We included an abbreviated version of Plutchik and Van Praag's (1986) scale to measure this.

Voluntary agencies

This part of the questionnaire focused on what the adolescents knew about voluntary agencies and helplines. It included questions about how they felt the services could be made more attractive and accessible to young people.

Prevention of self-harm and improvement of the local environment

In the final section of the questionnaire, the adolescents were asked two open-ended questions. The first concerned what they thought could be done to prevent young people from feeling like they wanted to harm themselves, while the second concerned how they thought life could be made better for young people in their neighbourhood. Responses to these questions provided a rich source of information about the adolescents' views. This section also provided an opportunity for adolescents who had not self-harmed (and who were therefore likely to complete the questionnaire more quickly than the adolescents who had) to spend time completing these questions so that there would not be an obvious time difference for completion of the questionnaire between them and the other adolescents. This reduced the risk of adolescents being able to work out who had self-harmed and who had not and kept them all occupied for the entire session.

Testing the questionnaire

The draft questionnaire underwent three pilot phases. In the first phase, we checked that pupils could complete the questionnaire in the space of a single school lesson. Pupils from a comprehensive school in London completed the questionnaire successfully within the constraints of the lesson time.

The second test run was completed by a high-risk sample of adolescents with psychiatric problems. Many from this sample had engaged in self-harm. We wanted to ensure that such a sample could also complete our questionnaire successfully. This proved to be the case.

Finally, having established that the questionnaire length was suited to completion within one lesson by both 'normal' and 'troubled' adolescents, we ran a focus group in a school in Oxfordshire with a mixed-ability group of pupils. The aim of the focus group was to check the readability of the questionnaire. In other words, we wanted to check that the adolescents could understand the terms and questions that were used. In addition, we wanted to find out whether they thought there were any other important questions we should include.

These three test runs provided us with valuable information that enabled us to refine the questionnaire into its final form for the study.

Sample of school pupils

Having decided upon our style of study and the tool to collect the data, we needed to work out how many pupils we would need to include in the study to ensure that our findings would be meaningful. We decided to aim to include a minimum of 5000 individuals. This number was based on a postulated prevalence of deliberate self-harm of 4 per cent, which was a conservative estimate made on the basis of the survey of the findings of previous studies from other countries (Evans *et al.*, 2005a). This sample size of pupils determined the number of schools that we needed to include in our study. In the event, as will be seen later, we were able to include a larger number of pupils in the study, the total number being 6020.

The most pragmatic method for investigating a representative range of adolescents is to choose a representative range of schools to be included in the study. The criteria we used to select the schools were:

- type of school attended (e.g. comprehensive, grammar or independent)

- single-sex and mixed

- range of ethnic backgrounds of pupils

- educational attainment of the schools (i.e. percentage of pupils attaining five or more GCSEs[1] at grade C or above)

- deprivation of the pupils (i.e. percentage of pupils entitled to free school meals)

- size of school.

We approached schools in Oxfordshire, Northamptonshire and Birmingham. The schools were chosen using the criteria outlined above to ensure that a representative range of school types were included. We selected the first appropriate school from the local list, contacted the head teacher by telephone and explained the purpose of our study. If a school declined to take part, we approached the next matched school on the list. The two most common reasons offered by staff at schools that declined to take part were that they had recently taken part in other research projects and did not want the pupils to lose any more teaching time, and that they had a school inspection (Ofsted[2]) looming, which they felt they needed to concentrate all their efforts on preparing for. However, the staff at these schools were generally very interested in our study and were keen to be updated on its progress.

If the head teacher expressed interest in their school being involved in the study, we sent them an information pack, which included a brief question-and-answer sheet, a sample consent form and a copy of the questionnaire. We then arranged a face-to-face meeting to discuss further the

---

1   A national educational qualification in England and Wales.
2   The Office for Standards in Education (Ofsted) is a non-ministerial government department whose main aim is to help improve the quality and standards of education and childcare through independent inspection and regulation and to provide advice to the Secretary of State for Education and Skills.

proposed inclusion of the school. Overall, 41 schools were included in our study. This took place in the spring and autumn terms of 2000 and 2001.

Absenteeism

When conducting school-based surveys of this kind, an important subgroup of pupils will inevitably be excluded, namely those who are absent on the day of the survey. These pupils will include those who are involved in prearranged out-of-school activities, those who are unwell, and those who are truanting (being absent from school without permission). Truants tend to have higher rates of problematic behaviours and so may be at increased risk for engaging in suicidal behaviour (Bagley, 1992; Grossman *et al.*, 1991; Roberts *et al.*, 1997; Yuen *et al.*, 1996). Also, among pupils who are absent due to illness, some will have psychological problems and may be at increased risk of deliberate self-harm. Excluding both groups of pupils brings with it the danger that the data collected will provide an under-estimate of the true number of adolescents who have engaged in deliberate self-harm. In spite of this, many school-based studies have done very little to address this potential source of sample bias. Indeed, some investigators have not mentioned the problem of absentees at all. Others have acknowledged the potential for bias that can result but have not indicated whether or how they have addressed the problem (e.g. Bensley *et al.*, 1999; Edman *et al.*, 1998; Hovey and King, 1996). Some researchers have simply called for future surveys to work with schools in order to follow up and include as many absent students as possible at a later date (e.g. Evans *et al.*, 1996; Olsson and Von Knorring, 1999).

A few investigators have attempted to explore the profiles of absentees compared with those of pupils who were present on the day the study took place (e.g. Fergusson and Lynskey, 1995; Galaif *et al.*, 1998). We designed a form that would be completed on the day of the survey to collect information about the absentees. We noted how many pupils of each gender were absent and whether the number of absentees was typical for the class. We also recorded the reason for absence if known. Finally, we reviewed the subsequent academic progress of a subgroup of these absentees.

Issues of consent

Several studies have explored the impact of using active or passive consent procedures regarding inclusion of adolescents in research where parental consent is required (e.g. Anderman *et al.*, 1995; Dent *et al.*, 1993; Kearney *et al.*, 1983). Active consent involves inviting parents of potential participants to opt in to the research. Under passive consent, there is an assumption that all parents of potential participants will be agreeable to their son or daughter taking part in the research unless they explicitly opt out. Obtaining active consent from parents of school pupils requires considerable effort from the potential participants themselves and, as such, often results in small and biased sample sizes. For example, Kearney and colleagues (1983) reported that a requirement for active written parental consent for pupil participation in a questionnaire survey focusing on drugs and alcohol produced a sample that was approximately half the size of the potentially eligible population. Such a high attrition rate suggests that in samples where active parental consent is required, selection bias is a strong possibility and it is, therefore, likely that only those participants who are particularly motivated or interested in the study will reply. This is likely to produce misleading results. In addition, Dent and colleagues (1993) concluded that pupils who were excluded from research studies as a result of parents not actively giving consent were at higher risk for a number of health and social problems. In addition, Layte and Jenkinson (1997) noted that individuals with higher levels of education and from higher social classes were more likely to respond to a call for active consent. The findings of both studies clearly highlight that it is practically impossible to obtain a representative sample of adolescents using the opt-in approach.

In the light of the above, we employed an opt-out (passive consent) approach to recruiting pupils from the schools. Some of the pupils we were targeting were aged under 16 years (the age at which a person is deemed to be capable of giving their informed consent). Once a school had agreed to take part, all the parents of the targeted pupils were written to and the purpose and procedures of the research were outlined. The parents were asked to notify the researchers if they objected to their child taking part in the research. This practice conforms to the British Educational Research Association (1992) guidelines, which suggest that schools act *in loco parentis* and therefore decide whether the proposed research is appropriate, whether it is necessary to inform parents and, if so, whether to enable parents to opt out. This approach towards dealing with sensitive matters conforms to general practice within schools in England (e.g. the issue of sex education is handled similarly).

How we implemented the study

Once a school had agreed to take part in the survey and a survey date had been arranged, all parents of the year group we were targeting were contacted by letter. We did not want to depend on the pupil's delivering the letters, and so we sent the school stamped letters to post out to the parents on our behalf. If a parent did not want their child to take part, they completed an opt-out sheet and sent it to the research team using a stamped addressed envelope that we had provided. In our study, the parents of only 139 pupils opted out of the research. Upon receiving a completed opt-out form, a note was made of the pupil's name, so that on the day of the survey we could ensure that they did not complete the questionnaire. We also arranged with the school for teachers to explain the purpose of the survey to all the pupils two weeks beforehand.

On the day of the survey, the research was again explained to the pupils. We used a script to ensure that as far as possible this procedure was standardised. The pupils were given the opportunity to ask questions and were also given the choice of opting out; only 23 pupils did so.

When explaining the questionnaire to the pupils, we made it clear that there were no 'right' or 'wrong' answers. We also explained that it was not a test and that we were really interested in finding out about how school pupils feel and cope with problems. We also made it clear that no information would be passed on to their teachers, their parents or their friends. Alternative activities had been arranged in advance for those pupils whose parents had opted them out of the study and for those who opted out themselves.

We found that of the few parents who chose to opt their sons or daughters out of the research, not all told their children that they had done so. Clearly, this could have been potentially upsetting for the individuals concerned. Therefore, care was taken when identifying the pupils whose parents had opted them out, to ensure that the situation was handled sensitively.

In most schools, the survey was conducted in the classroom, although some schools arranged for the sports hall to be available so that the whole year group could participate at the same time. We encouraged teachers to stay in the background as we thought that this would help reassure the pupils about the confidential nature of the survey. Pupils were sat as far apart from each other as the dimensions of the room would allow. The private nature of the questionnaire was emphasised, and all participants were asked to complete it in silence. In the early stages of completing the questionnaire, some pupils made jokes, for instance about who had drunk the most alcohol, but once they began to answer the more serious questions focusing on life events, pupils quietened down and concentrated on the business of answering the questions in silence. As a team, we were impressed by the serious manner and level of maturity demonstrated by most of the pupils who took part in our study. Informal conversations with the groups afterwards showed that the adolescents liked the fact that they were being asked for their opinion on such important topics. While the pupils were completing the questionnaire, the researchers collected data from the teachers concerning absentees.

Safety-net arrangements

We were aware that the process of completing the questionnaire could result in some individuals identifying themselves as 'having problems'. Also, it was possible that the process of asking questions of a sensitive and personal nature might have caused distress. Therefore, all the research team members underwent training that would enable them to deal with situations in which pupils disclosed their problems. In addition, during the initial meeting with the school, arrangements were made to inform the school welfare representatives and to prepare them for the possibility that pupils might seek their help in the days following completion of the questionnaire. Also, once all the pupils had completed the survey, a sheet listing useful contact details was handed out to all pupils. This sheet outlined the different options available to pupils if they were experiencing problems, highlighting the role of GPs and also focusing on a number of helplines that were relevant to the issues that had been raised by the questionnaire. This information sheet is shown in Appendix II. For some schools, the information sheet also indicated specific sources of help that the school staff wanted to be included, e.g. information about a specific staff member who could provide confidential help.

Summary

In this chapter, we have described the methodological issues that we considered and addressed when planning how to collect the data for our school-based study to determine the prevalence of deliberate self-harm and related phenomena among the adolescent population. We have explained the rationale behind our planning of the project, how we decided on our approach, and how we developed, tested and then implemented our schools study, including the reasons for using an anonymous self-report questionnaire. We have described the content of the questionnaire, which included questions about sociodemographic characteristics of the pupils, about smoking, alcohol and drug use, and about stressful events and problems that the adolescents may have faced. We asked about acts of deliberate self-harm and thoughts of self-harm in a very careful way, including obtaining descriptions of episodes of self-harm that allowed us to see whether these met our study criteria and also to report on the different types of method used.

We used a standardised method for investigating motives underlying acts of self-harm. Adolescents who had engaged in acts of self-harm were asked about whether they had tried to get help before or after and the source of the help. They were also asked whether they had gone to hospital as a result of the act. All the pupils were asked whether they had thoughts about harming themselves but had not actually done so and, if so, whether they had sought help. They were also asked about what types of coping strategy they used when facing difficult situations.

We assessed a range of psychological characteristics using standardised questionnaires. These characteristics include depression and anxiety, self-esteem and impulsivity. The pupils were asked about their knowledge of telephone helpline services and whether these could be made more attractive to adolescents. Finally, the pupils responded to two open-ended questions about what might help prevent adolescents from feeling that they wanted to harm themselves, and how life could be made better for young people in their neighbourhood.

We then described how we tested out the questionnaire before the study began, how we chose the sample of schools so as to make it as representative as possible of adolescents in England, how we dealt with the problem of absentees on the day of the survey, and what we did to ensure both parental and pupil consent to inclusion in the study. Finally, we described the practical arrangements for carrying out the survey, including what we did to try to ensure that pupils who identified themselves as having problems could get help. In the next chapter, we describe our findings on the size of the problem of deliberate self-harm among the adolescents who took part in our study.

CHAPTER 3

The Nature, Prevalence and Impact of Deliberate Self-harm and other Suicidal Phenomena in Adolescents

Introduction

This chapter focuses on the extent and nature of deliberate self-harm and other suicidal phenomena in adolescents. We report the findings from our schools study and then consider the international evidence on this topic. The methods used in acts of deliberate self-harm are described, together with the motivation or stated intention behind such acts. We also consider the extent of premeditation involved and repetition of self-harm. The frequency with which hospital presentation results from self-harm is examined, including the factors associated with this outcome. Finally, we explore the impact that self-harm and suicide have on family members and friends.

Deliberate self-harm

As mentioned in the previous chapter, adolescents in our schools study were asked to indicate whether they had harmed themselves intentionally, such as by taking an overdose or trying to harm themselves in any other way. If they answered positively to this question, they were then asked a number of questions about the last time that they had harmed themselves in order to provide us with a greater understanding of their experiences. Adolescents reporting an act of deliberate self-harm were also asked to describe the act. Those adolescents who had deliberately tried to harm themselves on more than one occasion were asked to describe the most recent episode. This not only allowed us to determine whether their description matched our criteria for deliberate self-harm but also enabled us to gain a greater understanding of the methods that adolescents employ when they engage in deliberate self-harm. We discuss these methods in greater detail later in this chapter.

Not all of the adolescents who reported that they had deliberately harmed themselves provided a description of what they had done. Others wrote that they did not wish to give details of their self-harm episode, some indicating that it would upset them too much or that they were too ashamed to write down what they had done. In all of these cases, we recorded that no deliberate self-harm information had been given and excluded them from the 'deliberate self-harm' category in subsequent analyses to be sure that we were including only those who had definitely engaged in self-harm.

As we noted in Chapter 2, other studies generally have not used such strict criteria – investigators have simply asked whether participants had engaged in deliberate self-harm or attempted suicide and accepted their responses at face value. Our approach enabled us to exclude cases that did not conform to our definition. For example, if respondents wrote that they had threatened to engage in self-harm but implied that they did not go through with the act, then these descriptions were recorded as not self-harm.

A total of 6020 adolescents took part in our schools study. Of these, 5293 completed all the questions on deliberate self-harm. A total of 13.2 per cent (784) adolescents reported having deliberately tried to harm themselves at some point in their lives. Deliberate self-harm *in the past year* was reported by 8.6 per cent (509) of adolescents. When our study criteria were applied, this figure dropped to 6.9 per cent (398 adolescents) (Table 3.1).

Table 3.1 Prevalence of deliberate self-harm in our schools study

	Self-report (%)	Meeting study criteria (%)
Past year	8.6	6.9
Lifetime/ever	13.2	10.3

Deliberate self-harm within the previous year was far more common in females than in males (11.2% v. 3.2%). Gender differences are discussed in more detail in Chapter 4 but are summarised in Table 3.2.

Table 3.2 Prevalence of deliberate self-harm in our schools study, by gender

	Self-report (%)		Meeting study criteria (%)	
	Males	Females	Males	Females
Past year	4.4	13.4	3.2	11.2
Lifetime/ever	7.0	20.2	4.8	16.7

Almost 100 adolescents did not answer the question about whether they had tried to deliberately harm themselves in some way. There are a number of different explanations for this, each of which has different implications for the likelihood that these adolescents had engaged in self-harm. For example, some adolescents may have accidentally turned two pages of the question-naire at once, thereby missing out this question, while others may have engaged in self-harm but found the question too difficult to answer. When we introduced the survey, we informed participants that they could leave out any questions that they felt were too difficult or painful to consider. Simi-larly, of those adolescents who responded positively to the question about self-harm, 22 per cent did not provide a description of what they did and were, therefore, excluded from the deliberate self-harm category because we were unable to determine whether their self-harm episodes met our criteria. However, while the prevalence figure of 6.9 per cent (deliberate self-harm in the past year meeting study criteria) is therefore likely to be an underestimate of the true prevalence, we can be confident that this included only definite cases of self-harm. While some readers might question the accuracy or even honesty of the adolescents' responses, their descriptions of the acts of self-harm conveyed a definite impression that the responses largely repre-sented actual behaviour.

In our review of the literature (Evans *et al.*, 2005a), only two other studies had enquired specifically about deliberate self-harm within the past year (Beebe *et al.*, 1998; Rubenstein *et al.*, 1989). These studies were both conducted in the USA and the overall prevalence figures were considerably higher (20% and 32%; respectively) than that reported in our study. However, these studies included relatively few adolescents (368 and 300, respectively) and had poor response rates. It is also unclear whether the sampling methods used were likely to result in representative samples, making comparisons with the results of our study unreliable.

In seven other studies (five from the USA/Canada and two from Australia), adolescents were asked whether they had engaged in deliberate self-harm at any time during their lives (a lifetime prevalence figure) (Allison *et al.*, 1995; Bagley, 1992; Brindis *et al.*, 1995; Conrad, 1992; Joffe *et al.*, 1988; Pearce and Martin, 1993; Pilowsky *et al.*, 1999). On average, the lifetime prevalence of deliberate self-harm was 14 per cent. This figure is very similar to that from our study (13.2%) before we applied our criteria for deliberate self-harm.

From our review of the international literature on suicidal phenomena in adolescents, we found considerable differences in the reported prevalence of deliberate self-harm. The vast majority of such community-based studies have been carried out in the USA and Europe (excluding the UK). However, there is little consistency of findings even from studies from within the same continent. In the USA, for example, the lifetime prevalence of 'attempted suicide' has been reported to be as low as 3 per cent (Lewis *et al.*, 1988) and as high as 30 per cent (Dinges and Duong-Tran, 1994). These differences in prevalence rates may be a result of the different ways in which the samples of adolescents have been identified. For example, in several studies, adolescents from only one or two schools took part in the surveys, but no explanations were given about the selection process. In other studies, the researchers had not made it clear how or why specific school classes or adolescents from within the schools had been selected. It should be noted that although the schools in our study were selected to provide a representative range of types of schools, the prevalence of deliberate self-harm in the previous year meeting our study criteria varied considerably between schools: the figure for the school with the lowest prevalence was 1 per cent while the highest was over 18 per cent.

Differences in prevalence rates for suicidal phenomena in the studies included in our review of the international literature may have been the result of differences in survey methodology. As we discussed in Chapter 2, it has been argued that anonymous methods of collecting information are particularly suited to collecting sensitive information in adolescents. Some people who would admit anonymously to having thoughts of self-harm or to having engaged in deliberate self-harm might not do so if such an admission could lead to them being identified (Safer, 1997b; Shochet and O'Gorman, 1995).

Finally, there has been considerable variation between studies in terms of the questions asked to assess the prevalence of suicidal phenomena. In many studies, the terminology that was employed has not been reported by the researchers. Furthermore, in most studies, a clear description of what is meant by self-harm has not been given, but reliance has been placed entirely on the adolescents' interpretation of the question(s). The results from our study suggest that a proportion of adolescents may either misinterpret a general question about self-harm or not have a clear understanding of what self-harm is.

In order to address the problem of absentees at the time of our schools study survey, we first investigated whether the absentee rate on the day of the survey was unusual. In more than three-quarters of the schools for which this information was available, the rate of absenteeism was in keeping with the usual pattern. Second, we tried to determine how the absence of some pupils may have influenced the findings by repeating the survey in three schools with pupils who had been absent on the original survey day. Unfortunately, the majority of the absentees were absent again. In those who could be surveyed, the rate of deliberate self-harm was virtually the same as in the main study. Finally, when we compared all the absentees on the original survey day with those who were present, we found that the absentees had poorer general attendance rates, were more likely to be in receipt of free school meals and went on to do less well in their GCSE examinations. Therefore, it is likely that the absentees do represent an atypical group of pupils, but it is not possible to say definitively how their having been excluded from the findings influenced the overall results.

As noted in Chapter 2, our schools study was conducted as part of a collaborative study with five centres in Europe and one centre in Australia. Findings have been reported for Norway (Ystgaard *et al.*, 2003), Hungary Fekete *et al.*, 2004), Ireland (Sullivan *et al.*, submitted) and Australia (De Leo and Heller, 2004). The method used for assessing the prevalence of adolescents with a history of deliberate self-harm was exactly the same in all the centres. It is therefore particularly informative to compare the findings from the seven centres (Table 3.3). The figures shown in Table 3.3 are modified in that they have been adjusted for age across the centres in order to make them more directly comparable, because the numbers of adolescents of each age varied somewhat between the centres (as a result, the figures for England differ slightly from those shown earlier in this chapter). There is a striking similarity in the findings for five of the countries (England, Ireland, Belgium, Norway and Australia), especially for the percentages of girls with a past-year and lifetime history of self-harm. The figures for the boys differ a little more. However, the large female-to-male ratio in the findings is clearly present in adolescents in all the centres. The lowest rates of deliberate self-harm, especially in the girls, were in the Netherlands and Hungary. Relatively low rates of self-harm have been reported previously from the Netherlands for people of all ages (Grootenhuis *et al.*, 1994; Schmidtke *et al.*, 1996), but not for Hungary (Schmidtke *et al.*, 1996).

Table 3.3 Prevalence of deliberate self-harm in school pupils in countries participating in the Child and Adolescent Self-harm in Europe (CASE) Study, by gender.

Country	Deliberate self-harm meeting study criteria			
	Previous year (%)		Lifetime (%)	
	Females	**Males**	**Females**	**Males**
England	10.8	3.3	16.9	4.9
Ireland	9.1	2.7	13.5	4.9
The Netherlands	3.7	1.7	5.9	2.5
Belgium	10.4	4.4	15.6	6.8
Norway	10.8	2.5	15.3	4.3
Hungary	5.9	1.7	10.1	3.2
Australia	11.8	1.8	17.1	3.3

Figures adjusted for age across all centres

Attempted suicide

Attempted suicide has been investigated in research studies more commonly than deliberate self-harm, perhaps reflecting the fact that most research has been conducted in the USA, where more attention appears to be paid to suicide attempts than to acts that may involve non-suicidal motives. The most comprehensive study to have investigated attempted suicide is one from the USA. This community-based survey of youth behaviour – the Youth Risks Behavior Survey – which includes more than 10,000 adolescents, has been conducted by the Centers for Disease Control and Prevention on a regular basis since 1990. In 2004, one of the findings of the survey was that 8.5 per cent of participants had attempted suicide one or more times during the preceding year (Centers for Disease Control and Prevention, 2004). As noted above, the term 'attempted suicide' implies that the act was intended to result in death. Therefore, some participants who had committed acts of deliberate self-harm but without such suicidal intentions may have responded negatively to this question.

We are aware of 32 other survey studies that have investigated the prevalence of attempted suicide in the previous year (two from Australia/New Zealand, one from Africa, five from Europe and 24 from USA/Canada). Overall, the mean past-year prevalence of attempted suicide was 7 per cent (Evans *et al.*, 2005a). The lifetime prevalence of attempted suicide has been investigated in 60 studies (two from Asia, four from Australia/New Zealand, 15 from Europe and 39 from USA/Canada), and the mean prevalence figure was 10 per cent.

We did not ask whether the young people who took part in our study had 'attempted suicide', as the term deliberate self-harm, which is generally used more frequently in the UK, was chosen for this investigation. The term 'attempted suicide' implies that death (i.e. suicide) was the intended outcome, whereas deliberate self-harm includes a broader spectrum of behaviours, including those where death may not have been the intention. However, we did ask adolescents who responded positively to the question about deliberate self-harm whether they had wanted to die as a result of their behaviour. Of those adolescents that had harmed themselves in the past year, 45 per cent reported that they had wanted to die at the time of the act. A similar proportion of males and females described that this was their intention (40.8% and 46.5%, respectively). The motives or intentions underlying this behaviour are discussed in more detail later, including the interpretation of the findings concerning the 'to die' motive.

Thoughts of self-harm

In our schools study, 15 per cent of adolescents said they had thoughts about harming themselves in the past year but without actually engaging in self-harm. As with actual self-harm, this was much more common in females than males, with almost three times as many females than males (22.4% v. 8.5%) reporting thoughts of self-harm. By comparison, the overall mean figure for all other studies that we have identified was 19.3 per cent (Evans *et al.*, 2005a). One possible reason for the slight difference between the figure from our study and the average for other investigations is that the adolescents in our study were classified according to the most severe suicidal phenomenon that they reported; in other words, adolescents who had engaged in deliberate self-harm were not also included in the 'thoughts of self-harm' figure – this was not always the case in other studies.

Whether adolescents had entertained thoughts of self-harm but not actually acted on these thoughts was also assessed in the countries involved in the CASE study. The proportion of girls who had had such thoughts in the previous year varied between the seven countries involved in the study, from 13.7 per cent in the Netherlands to 36.6 per cent in Hungary; for boys, the proportions varied between 5.6 per cent in the Netherlands and 17.9 per cent in Hungary. The findings for the other five countries (England, Ireland, Belgium, Norway and Australia) were intermediate between those for the Netherlands and Hungary. The prevalence figures for thoughts of self-harm in adolescents in these five countries were very similar: between 25 and 32 per cent in girls, and between 8 and 14 per cent in boys. The possible explanations for the very different levels of these phenomena in the Netherlands and Hungary are discussed in the next chapter.

The relatively high prevalence figures for deliberate self-harm and thoughts of self-harm in adolescents in our schools study and in most other investigations that we have identified (Evans *et al.*, 2005a) suggest that such behaviour and/or thoughts may not always indicate severe pathology but for some adolescents may indicate a period of transient distress. Of course, in other cases, the thoughts or behaviours will reflect major and persistent distress, amounting to psychiatric disorder. In such cases, the risk of future serious suicidal acts, including possible suicide, will be high. Longitudinal studies in which groups (cohorts) of adolescents are followed up over time are required in order to determine the extent of risk of this; such studies are rare. An important example of this type of study was conducted in New Zealand by Fergusson and colleagues (2005a,b), who have been following a cohort of 1265 children (635 boys, 630 girls) born in 1977. The cohort has been studied at birth, 4 months, 1 year, annual intervals to 16 years and again at ages 18, 21 and 25 years, using information from a combination of sources, including parental interviews, teacher reports, psychometric testing, self-reporting and medical and police records.

Suicide threats and plans

In our schools study, the adolescents were asked whether they had ever told someone that they were going to harm or kill themselves but without actually carrying out an act of self-harm. Of the adolescents that responded to this question, 7.5 per cent said that they had done so. Although the prevalence of suicide threats was not investigated widely in the studies we included in our review, it is an important area for consideration. Suicide threats have been found to be linked to later suicide attempts and are a means by which suicidal intent is communicated to others, therefore providing potential opportunities for intervention. We know of four other studies, conducted in Australia (Allison *et al.*, 1995), France (Stork, 1972) and the USA (Cole, 1989; Kandel *et al.*, 1991), in which the lifetime prevalence of suicide threats was investigated (Evans *et al.*, 2005a). Compared with our study, similar proportions of adolescents in these studies were found to have made such threats.

We did not investigate the prevalence of suicide plans in our schools study. Nevertheless, such plans have been shown to be an important predictor of later suicide attempts (Kessler *et al.*, 1999). The prevalence of suicide plans has been investigated in several other studies, including 11 studies in which the prevalence in the past year was examined and 13 studies in which lifetime prevalence was assessed. On average, 12 per cent of adolescents said that they had made a plan for suicide within the previous year and 16 per cent said they had done so at some point in their young lives (Evans *et al.*, 2005a).

Methods used in acts of deliberate self-harm

In our study, the two most commonly reported single methods of deliberate self-harm in the previous year that met our criteria for deliberate self-harm were self-cutting (55.3%) and self-poisoning (21.6%) (Figure 3.1). In addition, self-cutting and self-poisoning in the same episode occurred in a further 5.8 per cent of acts. Other single methods included self-battery

(2.3%), consumption of a recreational drug with intent to cause harm (3.2%), jumping from a height (1.5%), burning (0.5%), hanging or strangulation (0.5%), ingestion of a non-ingestible substance or object (0.2%) and electro-cution (0.2%).

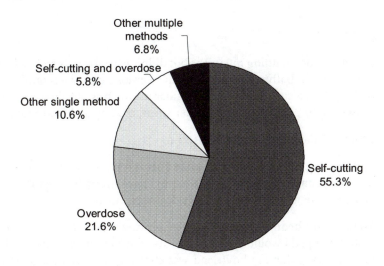

Figure 3.1 Methods of deliberate self-harm described by adolescents in our schools study who reported harming themselves in the previous year.

Some examples of adolescents' descriptions of their acts of self-harm are provided below to illustrate the nature of these acts.

Self-cutting

> I cut my arm repeatedly but did not cause any serious or lasting damage.

> I wanted to cut myself because I was angry. My mum was going through a separation and had just got together with someone new, who, within a few weeks was living with us. It wasn't bad cuts, just with a compass and a small piece of plastic. I have overcome that now.

> I felt really depressed – nothing seemed to be going well so I tried to slit my wrists but I didn't have the guts to do it. I felt so ashamed at my cowardice I took the razor blade and cut my arms instead – pressure to be thin and pretty – everybody else seems thinner, prettier and more confident.

I was very upset with who I was. I felt like everything I did was wrong and everything I was, was wrong. I felt like I wasn't good enough. To clean up the inside I used to make myself sick to make people love the outside. The pain was worse so I would cut myself with a razor. It was never a very bad cut; it was just a way of forgetting the pain inside.

Self-poisoning

I thought about cutting my wrists but didn't have the guts so I locked myself in the bathroom and took an overdose of paracetamol (13 tablets). I also suffer from trichotilamania which is an illness which causes me to pull my hair out under stress, anxiety and frustration.

I took 27 paracetamol and 30 aspirin.

I was having some trouble with some girls at school and I took at least 30 paracetamols (overdose). (Self-harm) I have strong feelings about a boy that I've just met and couldn't deal with them.

Went to my bedroom coz I was feeling down and took a load of tablets. I hoped I wouldn't wake up. I also felt a failure at school and I kept thinking that my boyfriend was cheating because he'd done it twice before and I also felt isolated.

I took a lot of pills – whatever I could find in the cupboard – and I took them. I didn't go to hospital and my parents were too busy arguing that they didn't notice.

I brought 2 boxes of paracetamol. I took 39 paracetamol and fainted. I nearly died and I was in hospital for 2 weeks; my kidneys failed and I had an operation.

Other methods

I hit a wall intentionally so I would break my wrist because I was angry and upset.

Ran out in front of lorry on the main road outside my house but best friend ran out after me and pushed me to the side.

I tried to strangle myself a couple of years ago with my school tie. I tried to do this as nothing was going my way, e.g. my schoolwork was suffering, I couldn't get a boyfriend and believed everyone hated me. I haven't tried to kill myself since!

Don't really know much about drugs but thought I could kill myself with ecstasy. My best friend had died. I wanted to be with her.

Tried to hang myself plus tablets – don't know what they were.

Ecstasy. It weren't funny.

Cut arm. Tried to strangle myself. Wanted to take overdose but couldn't find any tablets.

Burnt hands, cut arms.

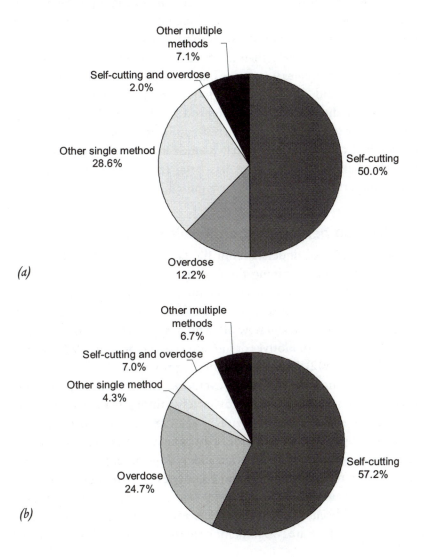

(a)

(b)

Figure 3.2 Methods of deliberate self-harm described by adolescents in our schools study who reported harming themselves in the previous year. (a) Males; (b) Females

Although most people described using only one method of self-harm, 12.6 per cent of those reporting self-harm acts in the past year that met our study criteria reported using multiple methods. The most common combination of methods was self-cutting and taking an overdose of medication, with approximately half of those who used multiple methods reporting doing both in the same act. This is in keeping with hospital-based studies of adolescents, such as that by Hawton and colleagues (2003b), in which 5.1 per cent of those presenting to hospital had carried out acts involving both self-poisoning and self-injury. Other relatively common multiple methods in our study included taking an overdose of medication with high levels of alcohol, and self-cutting combined with self-battery.

Females were more likely than males to have either cut themselves or taken an overdose, but males were more likely to report other single methods (e.g. self-battery) and multiple methods (other than overdose and self-cutting). These findings are shown in Figure 3.2. It is particularly interesting that although the research literature on self-cutting is focused almost entirely on females, half of the males who self-harmed in our study had cut themselves. This phenomenon in males has been rather neglected, probably because its importance has not been recognised.

The motivation behind deliberate self-harm

An important aspect of understanding the factors that lead to deliberate self-harm comes from examining the motives or intentions involved. One way to do this is to ask adolescents to explain their behaviour. However, this often results in diverse responses from very different domains, e.g. intent and specific problems. Another, and now often used, approach is to ask individuals to choose from a list of motives or intentions (Bancroft *et al.*, 1976, 1979; Hjelmeland *et al.*, 2002). The principal finding from a study of adolescents who presented to hospital following overdoses and in which the second approach had been used was that approximately a third said they had wanted to die at the time of the acts (Hawton *et al.*, 1982a). The most common motives chosen by the adolescents from a list of possibilities were to get relief from distress, escape from their situation and to show other people how desperate they were feeling. Boergers and colleagues (1998) obtained similar results in a study of US adolescents who had self-harmed. These studies have, however, all been confined to patients admitted to hospital as a result of self-poisoning. There are two limitations to this approach. First, exclusion of those who engage in deliberate self-harm but who do not go to hospital means that a large group of self-harmers from the general population is omitted. Second, since the focus of the hospital-based studies has been solely on those adolescents who take overdoses, our current understanding of the motives and premeditation involved in self-harming can be applied only to those who take overdoses and receive medical treatment.

Information on the motives of adolescents who engage in deliberate self-harm and who do not receive medical treatment, including those who choose methods other than overdose, will widen our understanding of what adolescents want to achieve through this behaviour. This can provide information that will assist in the planning of preventive initiatives. As will be seen later, it is also very relevant to the assessment and provision of aftercare for adolescents who have self-harmed.

In investigating the motives for deliberate self-harm in our schools study, we first asked adolescents to describe in their own words why they thought they had taken an overdose or had tried to harm themselves. This allowed them to spontaneously report their reasons for the act. The adolescents were then asked to choose from a list of eight motives those that explained why they had carried out the act. They could choose more than one reason if they felt that more than one applied. This list, as we indicated earlier, was adapted from that used by Bancroft and colleagues (1976, 1979). The proportions of adolescents who reported self-harm in the past year that met with study criteria and positively endorsed each of the eight motives are shown here:

- I wanted to get relief from a terrible state of mind – 72.8%.

- I wanted to die – 52.8%.

- I wanted to punish myself – 46.3%.

- I wanted to show how desperate I was feeling – 40.7%.

- I wanted to find out whether someone really loved me – 31.3%.

- I wanted to get some attention – 24.0%.

- I wanted to frighten someone – 21.1%.

- I wanted to get my own back on someone – 14.3%.

More females than males who had self-harmed endorsed each answer, except for wanting to frighten someone and wanting to get their own back on someone (Figure 3.3). The most marked gender differences were for getting relief from a terrible state of mind, using self-harm to punish oneself, and to find out whether someone really loved the person, each of which was endorsed more frequently by females.

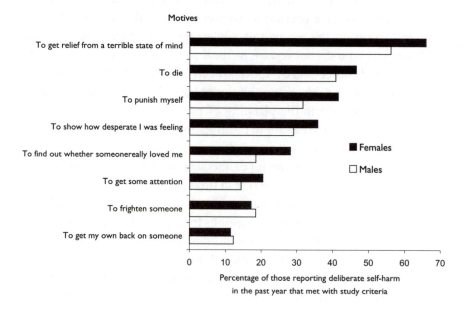

Figure 3.3 Motives for deliberate self-harm (DSH) reported by adolescents in our schools study who had harmed themselves in the previous year. From Rodham et al. (2004), with permission.

How did the motives that were chosen differ according to different methods of self-harm? As noted above, the two most commonly reported methods were self-cutting and self-poisoning. Because of the relatively small numbers and variable nature of the other methods of self-harm, we have focused on the differences in motives between the adolescents who took overdoses and those who cut themselves (Rodham *et al.*, 2004). Less than 1 per cent of those who cut themselves compared with more than 10 per cent of those who took overdoses mentioned spontaneously that they had wanted to die at the time they engaged in deliberate self-harm. In contrast, when asked to choose reasons from the list, many more respondents in each group chose 'wanted to die' (Table 3.4). However, those who took overdoses (66.7%) were more likely to indicate this motive than those who cut themselves (40.2%). The other difference between the two groups of adolescents' choices of reasons from the list was that those who took overdoses were more likely to say that they had wanted to find out whether someone really loved them (41.2% v. 27.8%).

Table 3.4 Comparison of motives chosen by self-cutters and self-poisoners in order to explain their acts

Motive chosen to explain act	Self-cutters % (n/N)	Self-poisoners % (n/N)	χ^2	P
I wanted to get relief from a terrible state of mind	73.3 (140/191)	72.6 (53/73)	0.01	0.91
I wanted to punish myself	45.0 (85/189)	38.5 (25/65)	0.8	0.36
I wanted to die	40.2 (74/184)	66.7 (50/75)	14.9	<0.0001
I wanted to show how desperate I was feeling	37.6 (71/189)	43.9 (29/66)	0.8	0.40
I wanted to find out whether someone really loved me	27.8 (52/188)	41.2 (28/66)	4.1	0.04
I wanted to get some attention	21.7 (39/180)	28.8 (19/66)	1.4	0.24
I wanted to frighten someone	18.6 (35/188)	24.6 (16/65)	1.1	0.30
I wanted to get my own back on someone	12.5 (23/184)	17.2 (11/64)	0.9	0.35

Not all the participants completed the different questions. Ns for each group are shown in brackets. From Rodham et al. (2004), with permission.

The most common reason reported spontaneously by the adolescents who engaged in self-cutting was depression:

Because I felt extremely low.

Depression and feeling horrible about myself and other people.

Depression, loneliness, self-pity.

In contrast, the most common reason reported spontaneously by those who took overdoses was escape:

Didn't want to live with problems any more; saw it as an easy way out.

Felt alone with no one to talk to so I thought it would be the only way to solve my problems.

I wanted to get away.

Only those who had engaged in self-cutting mentioned that they had done so because they were angry or wanted to relieve tension:

Because I was so angry at myself and it felt good while I was doing it as it felt like a release as if every cut I did was making it better.

Because I was upset and angry and to get all the hate out I cut myself a lot of times on my arm.

I think it helps me relax. I cut myself for the same reasons that I smoke. It calms me down. I used to scream and throw stuff, now I just bleed a little, but seriously it does help.

We also looked at gender differences in motives for self-harm in those who cut themselves and those who self-poisoned. In the males, there was no difference in the reasons selected between those who cut themselves and those who took overdoses. However, more of the females who had taken overdoses (66.7%) said that they did this because they wanted to die compared with those who cut themselves (42.4%). The girls who had cut themselves were also far more likely than the boys who did this to explain their self-harm episode by saying that they had wanted to punish themselves (51.0% v. 25.0%). The girls who cut themselves were also more likely than the boys to say that they were trying to get relief from a terrible state of mind (77.2% v. 60.9%). There were no differences between the boys and the girls who took overdoses in terms of the motives they indicated for these acts.

Premeditation

Studies of adolescents who have deliberately harmed themselves and presented to general hospitals have demonstrated that their behaviour is often impulsive – that is, it appears to have involved little apparent premeditation (Apter *et al.*, 1993; Hawton *et al.*, 1982a). For example, in a study of adolescents who had taken overdoses, 66 per cent said that they had had thoughts about the act for less than one hour beforehand (Hawton *et al.*, 1982a). A similar phenomenon has been shown in adults who have taken overdoses (Williams, 1997).

In our schools study, we asked adolescents about the length of time they had spent thinking about taking an overdose or harming themselves before they had actually implemented their plan. We found that 43.2 per cent had thought about it for less than an hour, while 13.1 per cent had thought about it for less than a day, 12.1 per cent for less than a week, 9.3 per cent for less than a month and 19.3 per cent for more than a month. We then compared the responses of those who had cut themselves with those who had taken overdoses and found that those who cut themselves were significantly more likely to have harmed themselves after having thought about it for less than an hour. It is much easier to engage in cutting oneself on the spur of the moment using whatever is at hand than it is to take an overdose, which requires a certain amount of planning. The latter may indicate more serious intent (i.e. wish to die). The shortness of the period of premeditation involved in many acts of deliberate self-harm (almost half of those who had cut themselves and over a third of those who had taken overdoses said they had thought about harming themselves for less than an hour beforehand) means that there is often little time for preventive intervention once planning has begun.

Repetition of deliberate self-harm

Just over half (54.8%) of the adolescents in our schools study whose descriptions of self-harm in the past year met the study criteria for deliberate self-harm said that they had harmed themselves on more than one occasion. Overall, this means that almost 4 per cent (216 adolescents) of the total sample reported multiple acts of self-harm. Males and females who reported deliberate self-harm in the past year were equally likely to have carried out multiple acts (56.8% and 54.4%, respectively).

Repetition of deliberate self-harm is common. It is highly important to understand more about the individuals who do this, as they are arguably in extreme distress. They are also known to be at particularly high risk of further self-harm and of completed suicide (Zahl and Hawton, 2004).

Findings from hospital-based studies show somewhat lower but nevertheless relatively high rates of repetition of self-harm. In adolescents aged
between 12 and 18 years who presented to the general hospital in Oxford
between 1990 and 2000 following deliberate self-harm, a third (34.7%) had
a known history of previous episodes (irrespective of whether these had
resulted in presentation to hospital). Similar proportions of girls (35.2%) and
boys (32.7%) had a history of a previous episode (Hawton et al., 2003b).
Some 10–15 per cent of adolescents presenting to hospital following deliberate self-harm will carry out a further self-harm act within a year and
re-present to the same hospital (Hawton et al., 1982c; Hawton and Fagg,
1992). On the basis of the findings from our schools study it is clear that this
repetition rate would be far higher if it were possible to include those adolescents who repeated self-harm but did not re-present to hospital.

A history of deliberate self-harm is the strongest predictor of whether
future repetition is likely after a current episode (Sakinofsky, 2000). Other
factors that have been found to be associated with repetition in adolescents include alcohol or drug misuse, long-term problems together with
behavioural disturbance, psychotic disorders, personality disorder, chronic
medical conditions/illnesses and not living with parents (Hawton et al.,
1982c; Headlam et al., 1979; Reith et al., 2003; Stanley and Barter, 1970;
Vajda and Steinbeck, 2000). A history of sexual abuse may also be relevant
(Vajda and Steinbeck, 2000). Further evidence regarding repetition comes
from an interview study of 45 adolescents who had presented to hospital
following deliberate self-harm (Hawton et al., 1999b). Repeaters at the time
of presentation had poorer scores than non-repeaters on measures of depression, hopelessness, trait anger, self-esteem and effectiveness of problem-
solving. When a multivariate analysis was conducted, level of depression
appeared to be the main factor associated with being a repeater. Depression
was also the key predictor of future repeats over the subsequent 12 months.

Hospital presentation

Presentation to a general hospital after deliberate self-harm was reported by
only 50 (12.6%) of the adolescents in our schools study who had engaged in
a self-harm act in the previous year (Hawton et al., submitted). Deliberate
self-harm is, therefore, clearly far more common in adolescents than repre-
sented by hospital presentation statistics. Thus, deliberate self-harm in adolescents can be likened to an iceberg, in which by far the largest proportion

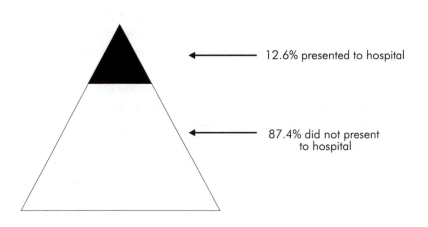

Figure 3.4 Iceberg model showing the percentage of adolescents in our schools study who reported presenting or not presenting to hospital following their most recent act of deliberate self-harm

of acts, which may be largely invisible to health professionals, do not come to medical attention (Figure 3.4).

In our study, hospital presentation was clearly related to method of deliberate self-harm. Using self-cutting as the reference category, hospital presentation was significantly more common in those who took overdoses, in those who used other single methods (such as attempted hanging or jumping) and where the deliberate self-harm method involved multiple methods (e.g. overdose and self-cutting). Slightly more of the boys than girls who had engaged in self-harm presented to hospital (14.7% v. 12.3%), possibly reflecting the trend for males to use more violent/dangerous methods of self-harm.

Hospital presentation was also associated with whether the adolescents had sought help from members of their families before deliberate self-harm. Those who said they had sought help were more likely to have presented to hospital. This may have reflected the degree of seriousness of their problems and/or that such adolescents were more willing to discuss problems with family members, including telling them when they had harmed themselves. However, this applied to only a minority of the adolescents who harmed themselves, since only just over one in ten of them said they had sought help from their family before engaging in deliberate self-harm and only a third of these had subsequently presented to hospital.

In the UK, self-poisoning with analgesics, especially paracetamol (acetominophen in the USA), has become a major problem. In adolescents who presented to the general hospital in Oxford between 1990 and 2000 after taking overdoses, approximately 60 per cent had taken paracetamol, in either pure or compound form (Hawton *et al.*, 2003b). Paracetamol can be very dangerous in overdose, with the risk of severe liver damage, which can cause death (O'Grady, 1999). In our schools study, 56.6 per cent of those who said they had taken an overdose in the preceding year had used paracetamol, a figure very close to the proportion in hospital-based statistics. Worryingly, those who took paracetamol in overdose were no more likely to present to hospital than those who took overdoses of other substances.

Impact of deliberate self-harm

Self-harm by adolescents is likely to have major effects on other people, especially family members and friends. Most information on the impact of suicidal behaviours on others comes from studies of actual suicides of young people. In a US study of family reactions to adolescent suicide, Brent and colleagues (1993) found that both mothers and siblings of adolescent suicide victims were far more likely to develop episodes of depression in the first six months following the deaths than mothers and siblings of control adolescents (i.e. living adolescents from communities matched with those where the adolescents who died by suicide had lived in terms of average income, population density, and racial and age distribution, but with no occurrence of suicide in the preceding two years). Interviews with peers of the adolescents who died by suicide showed that their depressive reactions appeared to be akin to bereavement complicated by major depression, a diagnosis in the *Diagnostic and Statistical Manual of Mental Disorders* (DSM) classification system of psychiatric disorders (American Psychiatric Association, 1980; Brent *et al.*, 1994).

Longer follow-up of the siblings and parents of the adolescents who died by suicide demonstrated that the mothers tended to experience further new episodes of depression during the two years following the deaths; this was not found in the fathers. When siblings were followed up three years after the deaths they had a much higher risk of depression, post-traumatic stress disorder and other psychiatric conditions compared with the siblings of the controls (Brent *et al.*, 1996).

Epidemiological research from Denmark has shown evidence of a greater long-term impact of adolescent suicide on mothers than fathers in terms of development of psychiatric disorders. In addition, this research showed that the risk of suicide is increased in parents after the death of an adolescent son or daughter by suicide (Qin and Mortensen, 2003).

Very little information is available concerning the impact of adolescent deliberate self-harm or attempted suicide on parents. In the USA, Wagner and colleagues (2000) studied parents' emotional and verbal reactions to the suicide attempts of 23 adolescents. Most of the parents interviewed were mothers. They reported a mixture of responses, including anxiety, especially on discovery of the act, caring feelings and sadness. Hostility was also felt by at least half the mothers. Caring feelings were more likely where there had been no previous suicide attempts by the adolescent. Higher lethality (i.e. dangerousness) of attempts was associated with greater caring feelings and absence of feelings of hostility. The most common reaction reported by fathers after the attempts was that they thought they needed to be careful what they said to their son or daughter. Hostility was reported frequently, but caring and supportive reactions were also common in fathers. However, the number of fathers in this study was small.

The reactions of parents to deliberate self-harm or expression of suicidal thoughts are clearly likely to be very important, especially in terms of determining whether the parents can help their children to deal with the problems they are facing. The reactions of the parents are also important in therapeutic interventions, especially when these involve the family directly (e.g. family therapy). Further research is needed to find out more about how parents respond to deliberate self-harm, the factors that influence their responses, the impact of their response on the adolescents themselves, and how the responses might influence the provision, nature and outcome of any therapy that is offered. The quality of family relationships is also likely to affect compliance. Thus, when King and colleagues (1997) investigated compliance with treatment recommendations in US adolescents who had been hospitalised because of being suicidal, they found that the most dysfunctional families and those with the least involved/affectionate father–adolescent relationships had the least engagement with parent guidance/therapy.

Summary and implications

Self-harm is common in adolescents when studied at the community level. By far the most common method of deliberate self-harm reported by adolescents in our study was self-cutting. Hospital presentation following self-cutting was rare compared with after other methods of self-harm. The fact that a greater proportion of adolescents who had taken overdoses compared with those who had cut themselves had presented to hospital explains why, to date, those who have taken overdoses have been the focus of most studies of deliberate self-harm. However, more than three-quarters of the adolescents in our study who reported taking overdoses in the preceding year also did not present to hospital. This is a surprising and worrying finding. Furthermore, many of the overdoses reported by such adolescents included relatively dangerous substances, especially paracetamol.

In keeping with the findings of hospital-based studies of adolescents who have self-harmed by Hawton and colleagues (1982a) in the UK, and Boergers and colleagues (1998) in the USA, the reasons most frequently endorsed by the adolescents in our schools study suggested that many used deliberate self-harm in order to cope with distress. Less frequently, they also indicated motives concerned specifically with interpersonal difficulties (e.g. attempts to influence other people's behaviour) when trying to explain their own behaviour. Substantial proportions of both those who took overdoses and those who cut themselves in our schools study said they had wished to die, which is perhaps surprising given the relative infrequency of hospital presentation following the acts.

It is clear that there are some differences in the reasons why adolescents engage in self-cutting rather than taking overdoses, and vice versa, with more of the self-poisoners in our study indicating that they wanted to die, both spontaneously and in response to a list of eight possible reasons. Multivariate analysis confirmed that the wish to die was the main difference in motivation between the groups. The less frequent choice by those who cut themselves of the 'to die' motive is in keeping with deliberate self-cutting often being associated with tension reduction (Brain *et al.*, 1998), especially in those who cut themselves repeatedly (Walsh and Rosen, 1989). However, it should be emphasised that four out of ten of those who engaged in self-cutting did endorse the 'wish to die' motive. In addition, they were significantly more likely to have spent less than an hour planning their self-harm episode compared with those who took overdoses (Rodham *et al.*, 2004). It is much easier to engage in self-cutting on the spur of the moment using whatever is at hand than to take an overdose, which requires a certain amount of planning and may, therefore, indicate more serious intent.

It is interesting that there were no major differences between the males and females who took overdoses in the reasons they chose to explain their self-harm episodes. However, among those engaging in self-cutting, females were more likely than males to say that they had done so because they wanted to punish themselves and because they wanted to get relief from a terrible state of mind. This is in keeping with findings of studies of clinical samples of females who have cut themselves (e.g. Hawton, 1990; Shearer, 1994). Males who cut themselves have received far less research attention than females, and yet studies have indicated that as many males as females are seen in emergency departments for self-cutting in the UK (Hawton *et al.*, 2004; Horrocks *et al.*, 2003). The results of our schools study suggest that in adolescents, there are gender differences in the motivation for self-cutting.

For the clinician assessing adolescent self-harmers after overdoses or deliberate self-injury, the findings of our study and other research highlight the need to include exploration of motives for self-harm in their assessments. Gaining an understanding of the motivation can be important not only in providing a fuller picture of the nature of self-harm in individual cases but also in addressing prevention of future episodes. Thus, for example, when a specific motive for an act can be shared between patient and clinician, they can then look at how alternative coping strategies can be used in future if the patient is confronted by circumstances similar to those that preceded the recent episode.

The impulsive nature of self-harming behaviour (almost half of those who cut themselves and over a third of those who took overdoses had thought about harming themselves for less than an hour beforehand) means that there is often little time for intervention. In addition, the reasons for self-harm most commonly endorsed by the adolescents suggest that they are often trying to escape from an unbearable situation ('to get relief from a terrible state of mind' or 'to show how desperate I was feeling'). Prevention should focus on reducing the problems that lead to thoughts of self-harm and on helping young people to acquire alternative methods of problem-solving and recognising sources of help. This is something that might be implemented in schools through discussion or mental health awareness educational programmes. It might also be promoted through the media. Schools-based initiatives are discussed in detail in Chapter 6, and the potential for media-based initiatives is considered in Chapter 8.

Just over half of the adolescents in our schools study whose descriptions of their acts of self-harm met our study criteria said that they had harmed themselves on more than one occasion. A history of deliberate self-harm is the strongest predictor of whether future repetition is likely. It is highly important to learn more about the group of adolescents who repeatedly harm themselves, as they are arguably in extreme distress and are most at risk of future self-harm and completed suicide (Zahl and Hawton, 2004).

In this chapter, we have also highlighted the major effects that suicidal acts by adolescents can have on other people, especially family members and friends. Much of the information on the impact of suicidal behaviour in young people comes from studies of actual suicides. There is currently relatively little information on the impact of deliberate self-harm by adolescents on family members and friends. Further research is needed to explore not only the effects on family members and friends but also the impact that the reactions of family members and friends have on the adolescent self-harmers themselves. The findings of such research are likely to be influential with regard to the provision, nature and outcome of any therapy that is offered.

In this chapter, we have focused on the extent of deliberate self-harm and other suicidal phenomena in adolescents. In addition, the methods used in acts of deliberate self-harm have been described and compared with those from hospital-based studies of adolescents who have deliberately self-harmed. The motivation or stated intention behind the act of deliberate self-harm has been explored in depth. We have also considered the impact of deliberate self-harm and suicide on relatives and friends. In the next chapter, we will examine the characteristics that distinguish adolescents who carry out acts of self-harm, or who have thoughts of self-harm, from other adolescents.

CHAPTER 4

How Do Adolescents who Deliberately Self-harm or Have Thoughts of Self-harm Differ from other Adolescents?

Introduction

It is important to try to establish the factors that increase the risk of deliberate self-harm and the development of thoughts of self-harm and suicide in adolescents as a basis for the identification and development of prevention and treatment programmes. In this chapter, we describe the factors associated with deliberate self-harm and thoughts of self-harm by considering the results from our schools study of adolescents in England as well as the findings from other studies reported in the international literature.

Gender

In recent years, several organisations have identified the prevention of suicidal phenomena in young males as a priority. However, although completed suicide is more common in younger males than younger females, deliberate self-harm and thoughts of self-harm are much more common in young females. In our schools study, for example, reports of deliberate self-harm in the previous year that met our study criteria had occurred in 11.2 per cent of the girls, but only 3.2 per cent of the boys. Thus, deliberate self-harm was nearly four times as common in the girls. Similarly, 22.4 per cent of girls reported having thoughts of self-harm in the previous year compared with 8.5 per cent of boys, a ratio of 2.6 to 1.

The results from research that has been conducted in a number of countries suggests that this pattern is internationally consistent. In our review of the international literature, including 88 studies, the results of almost every study showed this gender difference. Thus, females were more likely than male adolescents to report suicide attempts, deliberate self-harm, suicide plans, and threats and thoughts of suicide and self-harm (Evans *et al.*, 2005b). Overall, the rates in females were at least 1.25 times greater than those in males, and for suicide attempts in the past year the prevalence for females was more than twice that for males. This is in keeping with the findings from studies of hospital admissions, in which the average rates of deliberate self-harm in adolescents are consistently higher in females than in males (Hawton *et al.*, 2003c; Kerfoot *et al.*, 1996; Schmidtke *et al.*, 1996).

Why should this be? There are several possible explanations, which are not mutually exclusive. One is that depression, a major factor contributing to self-harm and suicidal thoughts, is more common in female than male adolescents. There is strong evidence to indicate that this is the case (e.g. Collishaw *et al.*, 2004; West and Sweeting, 2003). In our schools study, the girls generally had markedly higher levels of depressive symptoms than did the boys. A second possibility is that the life stresses and problems likely to increase vulnerability to suicidal phenomena or precipitate thinking about deliberate self-harm occur more frequently in girls. In terms of vulnerability factors, experiences such as child sexual abuse, which are known to increase risk of suicidal behaviour, occur more frequently in girls than in boys. There is less evidence that acute stressors are more common in girls. However, young girls may be more vulnerable than young boys to the negative effects of, for example, break-ups of relationships with partners. Some other factors that contribute to self-harm, such as alcohol and drug abuse, are clearly more common in boys than girls. Another possibility is that boys readily use other more outwardly directed means of dealing with distress and anger, such as delinquent behaviour, fighting and other types of aggression, and are perhaps also more likely to use alcohol or drugs to smother bad feelings (although rates of alcohol abuse by young girls in the UK have risen markedly over recent years) (Boreham and Blenkinsop, 2004).

A further possible explanation is that deliberate self-harm serves somewhat different purposes in girls and boys, girls tending more often to use it as a means of communicating distress, to temporarily blot out bad feelings or for tension relief (especially self-cutting). There is some limited evidence to suggest that this is the case. For boys, self-harm may be viewed more in terms of actual suicide attempts. Finally, as will be seen later, girls may be more vulnerable to the contagious influences of self-harm by others.

Age

The majority of adolescents in our study were 15 or 16 years old. As the age range was so narrow, it would be impossible to identify accurately whether and how the prevalence of suicidal phenomena varies with age. The most informative way in which to investigate this would be to conduct a longitudinal study, in which the same individuals are surveyed over a number of years to look for trends over time. Two studies that we identified through our review of the international literature allowed trends according to age to be investigated in this way. Domènech and colleagues (1992) examined changes in the prevalence of suicidal thoughts with increasing age in Spanish adolescents. Suicidal ideation was assessed annually over a three-year period. The girls were evaluated from 11 to 13 years and the boys from 12 to 14 years. (The study was part of a larger project focused on pubertal development, which explains the difference in ages studied for the two genders.) For both males and females, there was no change in frequency of individuals expressing suicidal ideation according to age. In a longitudinal survey from the USA, adolescents were assessed annually over a three-year period (Garrison et al., 1991). At the beginning of the study the adolescents ranged in age from 11 to 15 years, with the majority (99%) being between the ages of 12 and 14 years. Suicidal ideation in this study was assessed using three items ('I felt like life was not worth living', 'I felt like hurting myself' and 'I felt like killing myself') and responses were recorded on a four-point scale ('Rarely or none of the time', 'Some or a little of the time', 'A lot of the time' and 'Most of the time'). A total score was obtained by summing the responses on these three items, with a possible range from 0 to 9. A score over 5 was classified as a 'high suicide score'. There were no changes in scores with increasing age. The results from these two longitudinal studies suggest that the prevalence of suicidal thoughts does not vary with age during early adolescence.

Longitudinal studies are by nature non-anonymous. As discussed earlier, perceived anonymity of a survey may well have an impact on the responses provided by adolescents. An alternative way to investigate the association between age and suicidal phenomena that would permit anonymity would be to compare children in different age groups or school years. Questionnaire surveys were employed in 30 of the studies identified through our review of the international literature (although not all were anonymous). In approximately half of these studies, a significant association with age was found. However, the direction of the association was not consistent: in some the prevalence of suicidal phenomena increased with age, whereas in others it decreased with increasing age. The age range of the samples varied considerably, which may account for the apparently contradictory findings. The results appear to suggest that there is a peak in suicidal thoughts and behaviours between the ages of 14 and 18 years. This is consistent with findings from hospital-based studies. In England, presentations for deliberate self-harm are rare in girls under the age of 12 years but increase steadily in frequency up to the age of 16 years and then remain at this level until the late teens (Figure 4.1). In boys, the pattern for onset of self-harm is similar, in that deliberate self-harm presentations start to occur in 12- to 14-year-olds, although at a much lower frequency than in girls; presentations then increase with each year of age, continuing to do so into the early twenties.

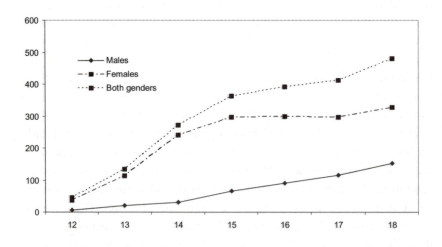

Figure 4.1 Frequency of deliberate self-harm by age and gender in 12- to 18-year-olds presenting to the general hospital in Oxford, 1990–2003. Data from the Oxford Monitoring System for Attempted Suicide.

Ethnicity

In our schools study, the prevalence of deliberate self-harm according to ethnic background of the adolescents was considered separately for males and females. Asian girls were significantly less likely to report self-harm than white girls. No significant difference in rates of deliberate self-harm between ethnic groups was found for boys. The finding regarding Asian girls is particularly interesting, since in the UK, deliberate self-harm has been identified as a significant problem in this group on the basis of hospital presentations (Merrill and Owens, 1986; Raleigh and Balarajan, 1992). Similarly, Bhugra and colleagues (1999) found that rates of self-harm in Asian women were one and a half times higher than those in white women. Furthermore, when age was taken into account, these differences became even more prominent, especially in the younger age group (between 16 and 24 years). In contrast, in a more recent paper it was noted that inception rates of deliberate self-harm among South Asian adolescents were no different compared with their white counterparts (Bhugra et al., 2003).

In our review of the international literature, the association between ethnicity and suicidal phenomena in US adolescents suggests that the prevalence of suicidal phenomena is higher in both Native American and Hispanic adolescents than in either black or white adolescents. This trend was found in the majority of studies in which this association was investigated and seemed to hold true for all suicidal phenomena (suicide attempts, deliberate self-harm, suicide plans, suicidal thoughts). This included the large National Youth Risk Behavior Survey (Centers for Disease Control and Prevention, 2004), in which higher rates of suicidal phenomena were found in Hispanic adolescents than either black or white adolescents, but with no differences between the latter two ethnic groups. However, in some of the studies the prevalence of suicidal phenomena did not appear to differ between ethnic groups. Significant differences tended to be reported only in the studies with relatively large sample sizes, suggesting that non-significant findings may be the result of inadequate power (i.e. insufficient numbers to detect a difference). However, there appears to be a general trend for suicidal phenomena (including suicide) to be more frequent in indigenous native populations (Brindis et al., 1995; Evans et al., 1996; Roberts et al., 1997).

One important factor to consider when looking at ethnicity is how ethnic groups are categorised. In many studies, adolescents from minority ethnic groups tended to be categorised as of 'other' ethnicity. The ethnicity of the minority will vary greatly from geographic area to geographic area, and it is important to be mindful of this when considering the generalisability of findings. This is especially so in view of research evidence that suggests risk of suicidal behaviour in ethnic groups is associated with population density. For example, Neeleman and Wessely (1999) found that in London, suicidal behaviour was more frequent in ethnic groups in areas in which they were in the minority than in areas in which they constituted a much larger part of the local population. Thus, the social experience of being part of a minority group may be an important factor. For example, prejudice and marginalisation may then be more common.

International differences

With regard to differences between countries, the results in our literature review suggest that the prevalence of suicidal phenomena is higher in the USA, Canada, Australia and New Zealand than in Europe, Mexico and Asia. Three studies attempted to investigate between-country differences in the prevalence of suicidal phenomena. Eskin (1995) compared the prevalence of suicidal behaviour in two countries, Sweden and Turkey, which differ considerably in a number of ways, including religion and social structure. There was no real difference in the lifetime prevalence of suicide attempts between the two countries. In the two other studies, however, differences were found. In one study, Mexican adolescents reported lower rates of suicidal thoughts than adolescents from the USA (11.6% and 23.4%, respectively) (Swanson *et al.*, 1992). In the other study, Russian adolescents appeared to be somewhat more likely to report suicidal thoughts and suicide attempts than Israeli adolescents (Ponizovsky *et al.*, 1999).

In Chapter 3 we noted the international findings from the Child and Adolescent Self-harm in Europe (CASE) study regarding similarities and differences in frequency of self-reported deliberate self-harm and thoughts of self-harm in adolescents (mostly aged 15 or 16 years). The use of precisely the same method of survey in all the centres and large sample sizes mean that comparisons between the findings can be made with confidence. The previous year and lifetime prevalence of self-reported deliberate self-harm meeting the strict study criteria were similar in England, Ireland, Belgium, Norway and Australia, especially for girls. Far lower rates of self-harm were found in the Netherlands and Hungary (see Table 3.3). However, in these countries, there were very different findings regarding the adolescents' reports of thoughts of self-harm. Adolescents of both genders in the Netherlands had the lowest rate of thoughts of self-harm of the seven countries in the study. This suggests that the levels of self-harm phenomena are generally low in adolescents in the Netherlands. By contrast, the frequency of thoughts of self-harm in Hungarian adolescents was the highest in the seven countries. This suggests that there are barriers to translation of thoughts of self-harm into actual acts. This could reflect differences in social attitudes to self-harm and availability of methods of self-harm. It is also possible that there are differences in the motives involved. For example, the Hungarian adolescents who had self-harmed, especially the girls, more often said that they had done this because they wanted to die, than did adolescents in other countries.

Psychosocial and health characteristics of adolescents who deliberately self-harm or have thoughts of self-harm

In considering the psychological and health factors that are associated with deliberate self-harm and thoughts of self-harm in adolescents, we have grouped them into five domains, each related to a specific area of life:

- mental health and well-being
- personal characteristics and experiences
- family characteristics
- experience of suicidal behaviour in others
- influence of the media.

Mental health and well-being
DEPRESSION AND ANXIETY

Levels of depression and anxiety were associated with suicidal phenomena in both girls and boys in our schools study. These associations appeared to be stronger for the girls than the boys, with both factors making an independent contribution (i.e. after statistically adjusting for associations with other factors) to the occurrence of deliberate self-harm in girls (Table 4.1) (Hawton et al., 2002). Not surprisingly, the association between depression and suicidal phenomena has been investigated in many community-based studies of adolescents. The findings from more than 25 studies from a number of countries provide conclusive support for such an association (e.g. Andrews and Lewinsohn, 1992; Fergusson and Lynskey, 1995; Meltzer et *al.*, 2001; Reinherz *et al.*, 1995). Furthermore, results from more complex multivariate analyses consistently indicate that depression is one of the factors most strongly associated with suicidal phenomena (e.g. Mazza, 2000; Pilowsky *et al.*, 1999; Rey Gex *et al.*, 1998). Hopelessness is a common symptom of depression, and it has been proposed that hopelessness may influence the relationship between depression and suicide intent in adolescents (Kazdin *et al.*, 1983). There is reasonable evidence in the international literature in support of an association between hopelessness and suicidal phenomena in adolescents at the community level, but it is unclear whether this association is direct (e.g. Allison *et al.*, 1995; Marcenko *et al.*, 1999).

In our schools study, it was notable that depression did not come out as one of the factors associated most strongly with deliberate self-harm when we applied more complex statistical analyses that took account of other factors, particularly in the boys (Table 4.1). This may be because the level of de-

Table 4.1 Associations between deliberate self-harm in the previous year and anxiety, depression, impulsivity and self-esteem in our schools study

	Males		Females	
	Odds ratio (95% CI)	P	Odds ratio (95% CI)	P
Depression	No association	No association	1.09 (1.03–1.15)	0.002
Anxiety	No association	No association	1.08 (1.02–1.14)	0.006
Impulsivity	No association	No association	1.10 (1.04–1.16)	<0.001
Self-esteem	0.84 (0.80–0.89)	<0.001	0.90 (0.86–0.94)	<0.001

Figures adjusted for a larger number of associations with other factors. CI, confidence interval; P, probability. From Hawton *et al.* (2002), with permission.

pression was assessed at the time the survey was conducted rather than at the time of self-harm. The difference between the results of our study and those of other studies in which a stronger association has been found may also be explained at least partially by the way in which depression was assessed. In our study, adolescents answered questions about symptoms of depression (White *et al.*, 1999) and were given a score that reflected the number and severity of symptoms experienced. In some other studies, depression has been defined using medical criteria, which identify individuals with clinical levels of depression and therefore include only those individuals with the most serious levels of depression. In our study, individuals with less severe depressive symptoms would also have been included in the analyses.

Evidence from research conducted in other countries indicates that anxiety and anxiety disorders (e.g. social phobia) are associated with suicide attempts and deliberate self-harm but may not be associated so strongly with thoughts of suicide. Anxiety disorders are relatively common in adolescents who present to hospital because of deliberate self-harm (Burgess *et al.*, 1998; Kerfoot *et al.*, 1996). Although symptoms of anxiety (e.g. agitation, sleep disturbance, sense of foreboding) may often be part of depressive disorders, there is growing recognition that anxiety disorders may influence the risk of suicidal phenomena. When Allgulander (2000) reviewed the literature on the association between anxiety disorders and suicidal phenomena in adults, he concluded that *severe* anxiety increases the risk for suicidal behaviour, both in its own right and especially when it exists along with other disorders. As anxiety is amenable to treatments, both psychological and pharmacological, suicide may be prevented by effective treatment of severe anxiety disorders.

IMPULSIVITY

In our schools study, we also found an association between our measure of impulsivity and deliberate self-harm. This seemed to make an independent contribution to risk of self-harm in the girls (see Table 4.1). In view of the emphasis on the contribution of impulsivity to risk of self-harm in general (Evans *et al.*, 1996; Mann *et al.*, 1999), it is surprising that it has not been investigated in any of the studies identified through our review of the international literature on community studies of suicidal phenomena in adolescents.

The concept of impulsivity is complex and potentially misleading. Superficially, impulsivity is generally regarded as a tendency to act on the spur of the moment. However, it seems likely that it results from a deficiency in problem-solving skills. When an individual who lacks problem-solving skills is faced by an apparently insurmountable problem and consequent distress, they may act rapidly by doing something that will provide immediate relief (including, possibly, deliberate self-harm). Thus, impulsivity may be a secondary phenomenon reflecting more general difficulties in coping.

SELF-ESTEEM

In our schools study, low self-esteem was also found to be one of the factors associated most strongly with deliberate self-harm and suicidal thoughts for both males and females. This was found even after taking account of a wide range of other factors (see Table 4.1). We are aware of five other community-based studies of adolescents in which the association between low self-esteem and suicidal phenomena has been investigated. The results also strongly indicate that recent or current low self-esteem is experienced by many adolescents with suicidal thoughts or behaviours (Fergusson and Lynskey, 1995; Marcenko *et al.*, 1999; Overholser *et al.*, 1995; Reinherz *et al.*, 1995; Simons and Murphy, 1985). This is perhaps not surprising as low self-esteem is a symptom of depression (Beck, 1967) and increases an individual's vulnerability to becoming depressed (McGee and Williams, 2000).

EATING BEHAVIOURS

Other mental health difficulties have been hypothesised as being associated with increased risk of suicidal phenomena. For example, sleep problems and feeling tired are common symptoms of depression and, unsurprisingly, both have been shown to be associated with suicidal phenomena in the few studies in which they have been investigated (Choquet and Menke, 1989; Gartrell *et al.*, 1993; Rey Gex *et al.*, 1998; Vignau *et al.*, 1997). In several studies, a significant association has been found in girls between suicidal phenomena and both poor body image and unhealthy eating behaviours. Whether there is such an association in boys is less clear. It is possible that the association between suicidal thoughts and behaviours and unhealthy eating behaviours is equally as strong for males as for females, but because there are fewer males with eating disorders it may be difficult to detect a significant association.

Surprisingly, the association between eating disorders meeting criteria for a psychiatric disorder and suicidal phenomena appears to have been investigated in only one community-based study, with mixed findings for female adolescents and non-significant results for males (Andrews and Lewinsohn, 1992). However, an association between suicide attempts and *eating behaviours* (e.g. avoiding eating when hungry) has been reported in three studies (Thompson *et al.*, 1999; Tomori, 1999; Wagman Borowsky *et al.*, 1999). A further two studies have investigated the association between suicidal ideation and abnormal eating behaviours. Kandel *et al.*, (1991) reported mixed results for males, but for females in this study all associations were significant. A strong association has been found between suicidal phenomena, low self-esteem and eating problems (especially bulimia) in studies of young people being treated by psychiatric services (McGee and Williams, 2000; Tomori and Rus-Makovec, 2000).

ANTISOCIAL BEHAVIOUR

We were unable to examine the role of antisocial behaviour and self-harm in our schools study because ideally this requires reports by informants other than the adolescents themselves. However, we did ask adolescents whether they had been in trouble with the police, and this was found to be associated significantly with deliberate self-harm, but not when other factors (e.g. mood, self-harm in friends and family, drug-taking) were controlled for. Various criteria, including specific behaviours and diagnoses, have been used to identify antisocial behaviours in other community studies. Overall, a significant and direct association between antisocial behaviour and self-harm has been found for girls, but the association in boys is less clear (e.g. Patton *et al.*, 1997; Reinherz *et al.*, 1995). Studies of adolescents who have died by suicide (Brent *et al.*, 1993; Houston *et al.*, 2001; Shaffer *et al.*, 1996) and adolescents presenting to hospitals following deliberate self-harm (Hawton *et al.*, 1982a; Kerfoot *et al.*, 1996) have indicated that both suicide and self-harm are linked strongly to antisocial behaviours.

DRUG CONSUMPTION

Drug use was identified as one of the stronger predictors of deliberate self-harm for both male and female adolescents in our schools study. Risk of deliberate self-harm was increased in adolescents who used any type of illicit drug (Figure 4.2). We also found that risk of deliberate self-harm was increased for each specific drug we asked about, namely hashish/marijuana/cannabis, ecstasy, heroin/opium/morphine, speed/LSD/cocaine and other drugs and substances (not including medication). An association between deliberate self-harm and drug use has also been found in several other studies (e.g. Bjarnason and Thorlindsson, 1994; Rossow and Wichstrøm, 1994; Wagman Borowsky *et al.*, 1999). The research evidence suggests that the association is stronger for hard drugs such as heroin and cocaine than for softer (and more widely used) drugs such as cannabis (e.g. Kienhorst *et al.*, 1990).

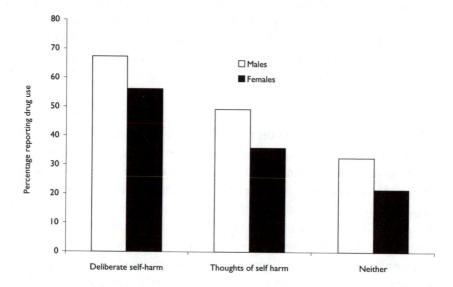

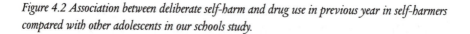

Figure 4.2 Association between deliberate self-harm and drug use in previous year in self-harmers compared with other adolescents in our schools study.

ALCOHOL CONSUMPTION

Alcohol consumption was also associated with deliberate self-harm in our schools study. The risk of deliberate self-harm rose with increasing amounts of alcohol consumed. For example, adolescents who reported drinking six to ten units of alcohol in a typical week had a 3.5-fold greater risk of deliberate self-harm in the year before the survey than those who said they never drank alcohol (Hawton *et al.*, 2002) (Figure 4.3). However, the analyses suggested that other factors mediated the relationship between alcohol use and self-harm.

Findings in the international literature provide additional evidence for an association between drinking and suicidal phenomena, and it appears likely that this association can also be a direct one (e.g. Bjarnason and

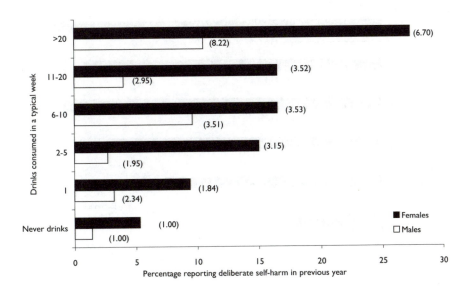

Figure 4.3 Association between deliberate self-harm and drug use in previous year and alchohol use in our schools study. Odds ratios for risk of self-harm compared with risks in those never drinking shown in brackets.

Thorlindsson, 1994; Rossow and Wichstrøm, 1994; Wagman Borowsky *et al.*, 1999). For attempted suicide, certain characteristics of alcohol consumption appeared to be predictive of an association, including especially high alcohol consumption and drinking strong alcoholic drinks, such as spirits (e.g. Choquet and Menke, 1989; Gartrell *et al.*, 1993).

SMOKING

Smoking was also associated with deliberate self-harm in our schools study. As with the consumption of alcohol, there was an incremental increase in risk of deliberate self-harm the more an individual smoked. Thus, boys who said they smoked 6–20 cigarettes per week were 3.25 times more likely to report deliberate self-harm in the preceding year compared with those who said that they did not smoke; in girls, the risk was increased 4.5 times (Figure 4.4). However, the association between smoking and deliberate self-harm did not appear to be a direct one. Our review of the international literature revealed several other studies in which an association between

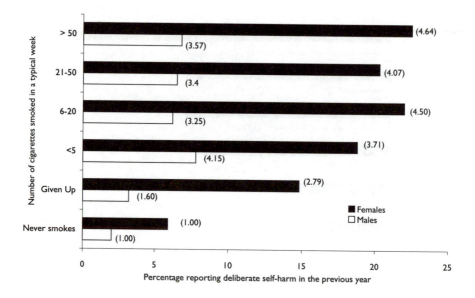

Figure 4.4 Association between deliberate self-harm in the previous year and smoking in our schools study. Odds ratios for risk of self-harm compared with risk in those never smoking in brackets.

smoking and both deliberate self-harm and suicidal ideas has been found, but again this association has usually appeared to be indirect (e.g. Bjarnason and Thorlindsson, 1994; Vannatta, 1996). It is unclear whether there are differences between the genders in this respect. Interestingly, the only study in which an association between deliberate self-harm and smoking was not found was conducted in Asia (Juon *et al.*, 1994), raising the possibility that cultural factors may be important in this regard.

Personal characteristics and experiences
SCHOOLWORK

Having problems keeping up with schoolwork was found to be significantly associated with suicidal phenomena in our schools study. However, due to the methodology we employed, we are unable to pinpoint whether struggling with schoolwork was one of the stressors contributing to deliberate self-harm, or whether adolescents who had self-harmed had disengaged from schoolwork, or whether self-harm and schoolwork difficulties both resulted from a third factor, such as low mood. Other studies have shown that several school-related factors appear to be associated with suicidal phenomena, namely poor academic achievement, poor school attendance, having a negative attitude towards school and schoolwork, and school misconduct (e.g. Bjarnason and Thorlindsson, 1994; Grossman *et al.*, 1991; Wagman Borowsky *et al.*, 1999). Some social activities, such as spending time in gangs and going to parties, have also been associated with an increased prevalence of suicide attempts (but not suicidal ideation) (e.g. Bjarnason and Thorlindsson, 1994; Wagman Borowsky *et al.*, 1999). It should be noted, however, that these findings are from relatively few studies.

As individuals progress through adolescence, the importance of peer relationships increases considerably. As will be discussed later, self-harm by friends is one of the key predictors of deliberate self-harm, but other aspects of peer relationships also appear to be important. Overall, the research evidence suggests that negative aspects of peer relationships, such as loneliness and breaking up with friends, increase the likelihood of deliberate self-harm (e.g. Bjarnason and Thorlindsson, 1994), but, surprisingly, positive aspects of peer relationships, such as degree of peer support, do not appear to offer protection against self-harm (Eskin, 1995). Having difficulty in keeping friends and having arguments with friends also seem to increase the risk of deliberate self-harm and suicidal thoughts.

BULLYING

Bullying occurs in all schools. Bond and colleagues (2001) noted that bullying can be considered to be a common and, as such, almost normal experience, but at the same time it is also an important cause of stress and physical and emotional problems. For example, Kumpulainen and colleagues (1999) found an association between involvement in bullying and a number of behavioural and psychological symptoms, including depression, anxiety, fear of going to school and low self-esteem.

Although the possible association between being bullied and the risk of suicidal behaviour has been recognised by adolescent psychiatrists (Rutter *et al.*, 1994), epidemiological studies have not usually investigated this. This is probably because the cross-sectional design of most studies means that it is impossible to determine causality. However, in a study of Finnish adolescents, Kaltiala-Heino and colleagues (1999) found that being bullied or being a bully was a sign that an adolescent was at increased risk of depression and suicidal behaviour. Similarly, in our schools study, being bullied was associated significantly with adolescent deliberate self-harm. Males who had been bullied were three times more likely to have engaged in deliberate self-harm than those who had not been bullied. Similarly, females were twice as likely to have engaged in deliberate self-harm if they had been bullied.

SEXUAL ABUSE

Adolescents in our schools study who said that they had been forced verbally or physically to engage in sexual activities against their will were at greater risk for deliberate self-harm compared with their peers. There was some evidence to suggest that sexual abuse may have been a slightly greater risk factor for self-harm for males than females. There is considerable evidence from other studies of adolescents for a strong and direct association between sexual abuse and suicidal phenomena. This is consistent with findings from other types of study (Chandy et al., 1996; Coll et al., 2001). Although most previous research has focused on sexual abuse in females, the effect (as the results of our study suggest) may be even more profound for males. For example, Choquet and colleagues (1997) found that 52 per cent of French males who had been raped had attempted suicide compared with 2 per cent of controls; for females, the comparable figures were 22 per cent of those raped compared with 12 per cent of controls. In addition, Darves-Bornoz and colleagues (1998) found that reactions to sexual assault differed by gender: females were more likely to be affected by medico-psychological symptoms, such as nightmares and somatic complaints, whereas males were more likely to express behavioural symptoms, such as repeated suicide attempts and substance misuse.

PHYSICAL ABUSE

In our schools study, we identified physical abuse as a factor that was associated directly with deliberate self-harm: adolescents who had experienced physical abuse were at least four times more likely to report deliberate self-harm compared with their peers. Some other studies have suggested a direct association between physical abuse and suicidal phenomena (Grossman et al., 1991; Wagman Borowsky et al., 1999). Straus and Kantor (1994) found that retrospective recall of corporal punishment during adolescence was associated with later-life suicidal ideation; however, other studies have not found such an association. For example, in South Africa, Flisher and colleagues (1997) found that physically abused children were no more likely to report suicidal thoughts and behaviours than non-abused children. It may be that the association is dependent on the severity of the suicidal phenomena, i.e. there may be an association with more serious suicidal phenomena, such as suicide attempts, but not with suicidal ideation. Differences in impact on suicidal phenomena may also depend on the identity of the abuser and the severity and duration of the abuse. Furthermore, serious abuse by parents may be associated with additional risk factors, such as family history of mental health problems and drug and alcohol abuse.

SEXUAL ORIENTATION AND BEHAVIOUR

Surprisingly, very few school surveys have focused on the possible association between suicidal phenomena and sexual orientation in adolescents. In our schools study, we asked the adolescents whether they had had any worries about their sexual orientation in the past year. Approximately 3 per cent of the sample reported having such worries. Females who were worried about their sexual orientation were four times more likely than females without such worries to report deliberate self-harm, and males with such worries were more than twice as likely as other males to report deliberate self-harm. In neither gender, however, was an independent association with deliberate self-harm found. This may well reflect the relatively low rate of reporting of these concerns.

In our review of the international literature, homosexual orientation in both genders and bisexual orientation in females were found to be associated with suicide attempts (Wagman Borowsky et al., 1999). This is in keeping with the findings from research on gay populations, in which a strong association has been reported (Herrell et al., 1999; van Heeringen and Vincke, 2000). In a review of the clinical and epidemiological literature, Bagley and Tremblay (2000) found elevated rates of suicidal behaviour in Canadian gay, lesbian and bisexual youths. Data from the larger surveys indicated that the risk for a serious suicide attempt is at least four times greater than for heterosexual adolescents. Depression, low self-esteem and experiencing suicidal behaviour in someone close have been identified as risk factors for suicidal phenomena in Belgian homosexual youths (van Heeringen and Vincke, 2000). Additional risk factors, such as rating homosexual friendships as less satisfactory (van Heeringen and Vincke, 2000) and homophobic persecution in schools (Bagley and Tremblay, 2000), have also been linked to the elevated rates of suicidal phenomena in homosexual youths.

In studies of young adolescents, having had sexual intercourse has been found to be associated significantly with suicidal phenomena (Benson and Torpy, 1995; Walter et al., 1995). Stress due to sexual activity has been shown to be related directly with suicidal thoughts and behaviours when stress due to other factors (e.g. family conflict, family and friend suicidality, achievement pressure) has been controlled for, indicating a direct relationship (Rubenstein et al., 1989). However, this conclusion is based on the findings from only one study and should, therefore, be treated with some caution. In our schools study, adolescents who had had serious problems with a boyfriend or girlfriend were also significantly more likely to report self-harm and suicidal thoughts than their peers who had not had such difficulties. This is in keeping with the high frequency of boyfriend/girlfriend problems found in adolescents who present to hospitals after deliberate self-harm, especially older adolescents (Hawton et al., 2003b).

Family characteristics

Overall, the risk of suicidal phenomena does not appear to reflect the socioeconomic characteristics of families of adolescents. However, two specific characteristics may be relevant, namely the father's level of education (Andrews and Lewinsohn, 1992; Dubow et al., 1989) and the adolescent being stressed or worried about their family's socioeconomic situation (Roberts et al., 1997). The absence of a clear socioeconomic effect is in keeping with the lack of a marked social class skew in adolescents attending hospital as the result of suicide attempts (Hawton et al., 1982b). This is in contrast to adults, in whom rates of attempted suicide are greatly elevated in lower socioeconomic groups (Hawton et al., 2003c; Platt et al., 1988).

Certain aspects of family structure appear to be linked to suicidal phenomena. In our schools study, female adolescents living with one parent were no more at risk of deliberate self-harm than those living with both parents. By contrast, males living with only one parent or with one parent and a step-parent were at greater risk for self-harm than males living with both parents. In the UK, after parental separation most children live with their mothers; based on this, it appears that living away from their biological fathers has a significant negative impact on males, increasing their risk for deliberate self-harm, but the impact on females is not so marked. As the risk for self-harm is still increased in males when living with a parent and step-parent, having adults of both genders in the household does not appear to mitigate against this effect. Other living situations, such as living with another relative or with a non-family member, were not associated with a significant increase in risk for self-harm, but this may have been because there were only a few individuals in such circumstances and so differences were not detectable. Interestingly, having parents who were separated or divorced was a significant risk factor for deliberate self-harm in both male and female adolescents.

The results of other studies have indicated that living apart from both parents can have a direct association with suicide attempts (Kaltiala-Heino *et al.*, 1999; Rey Gex *et al.*, 1998). There is some other evidence that parental divorce and the presence of a step-parent can be associated with suicide attempts and ideation (Andrews and Lewinsohn, 1992; Kaltiala-Heino *et al.*, 1999). There was also a suggestion in an American study of an association with absence of the adolescent's father but not with absence of the mother (Andrews and Lewinsohn, 1992). However, it may have been that too few adolescents were living apart from their mothers for any impact on suicidal phenomena to be detected. In a review, Kelly (2000) reported that divorce per se is not the major cause of problems during childhood, but that marital conflict is a more important factor. Many of the problems experienced by children in families in which parents subsequently divorce can be observed long before separation, and the intensity and frequency of conflict are predictors of child adjustment. Several studies suggest that conflicts and arguments within the home are associated clearly and directly with the prevalence of suicidal phenomena, whereas family harmony and cohesion appear to have a protective effect (e.g. Reinherz *et al.*, 1995; Stewart *et al.*, 1999; Wright, 1985). These associations appear to be stronger for females than for males.

For both male and female adolescents in our schools study, those who had argued or fought with their parents and those with arguing parents were at increased risk for both deliberate self-harm and suicidal thoughts. Other studies have shown that other aspects of the adolescents' relationships with their parents, in addition to family discord and cohesion, appear to be associated with suicidal phenomena. Thus, various emotional aspects of the relationship, such as lack of parental support and criticism from parents, also appear to be relevant (Eskin, 1995; Rubenstein *et al.*, 1989). Overall, the evidence indicates that this association is important for both male and female adolescents (e.g. Wagman Borowsky *et al.*, 1999). It is unclear whether the associations with other emotional aspects of the relationship between adolescents and their parents are direct. The results of one study indicated that along with poor general family functioning, too little or too much (i.e. over protectiveness) parental supervision can be associated with an increased prevalence of suicidal phenomena (Wagner *et al.*, 1995). Also, good communication with and feeling understood by family members appear to reduce risk (Stewart *et al.*, 1999; Wagner *et al.*, 1995).

Some studies have shown an association between having a parent with mental health difficulties and adolescent suicidal phenomena (e.g. Meltzer *et al.*, 2001), but, perhaps surprisingly, this relationship appears to be indirect (Joffe *et al.*, 1988; Rubenstein *et al.*, 1989). It is unclear whether drug and alcohol use by family members is associated with deliberate self-harm in adolescents, but the limited evidence available indicates that if a relationship does exist then it is indirect (Joffe *et al.*, 1988; Wagman Borowsky *et al.*, 1999). A family history of offending may also be relevant, but this has received limited research attention (Fergusson and Lynskey, 1995; Joffe *et al.*, 1988).

Experience of suicidal behaviour in others

One factor that was associated particularly strongly with deliberate self-harm in our schools study was having a friend who had recently self-harmed. For both males and females, this factor was one of the strongest predictors of self-harm. Males who had a friend who had engaged in deliberate self-harm were almost seven times more likely to engage in self-harm than males who did not have a friend who had self-harmed. Similarly, females were four and a half times more likely to engage in deliberate self-harm if they had a friend who had also self-harmed (Figure 4.5) This might be because pupils from schools with higher rates of deliberate self-harm may be more aware of adolescents who have harmed themselves. However, where the same comparison was made for the two genders separately, the association was found only in females. When the comparison was made according to the method of deliberate self-harm (self-cutting or overdose), the association was found only for females who had cut themselves. Thus, there may be a particularly contagious element to self-cutting behaviour that is confined to females. Unfortunately, we do not know what specific methods of deliberate self-harm were used by the friends.

Several other studies of adolescents, mostly from the USA, have also found evidence for such an association (e.g. Bjarnason and Thorlindsson, 1994; Wagman Borowsky *et al.*, 1999). In adolescents, the strong modelling influence of suicidal behaviours by peers is also shown by the clustering of suicides that can occur in this age group (Gould *et al.*, 1989, 1994). Possible explanations for these findings are discussed below.

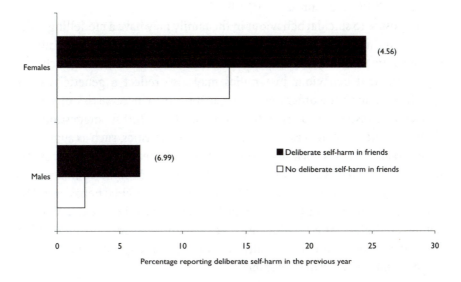

Figure 4.5 Association between deliberate self-harm in the previous year and having friends who had also engaged in deliberate self-harm in the previous year in our schools study. Odds ratios in brackets.

In our schools study, having a friend who had died by suicide was not found to be associated with deliberate self-harm. However, this may reflect the relative rarity of such events, and an extremely large sample of adolescents would be required to establish whether there is such an association. Alternatively, such an experience may give adolescents a greater understanding of the negative impact of suicide on others and may prevent adolescents from taking such a course of action themselves. Also, others may recognise that they have had a very difficult experience and may provide additional help and support, allowing adolescents to cope with their difficulties.

We found that self-harm by a family member was a strong predictor of deliberate self-harm. This finding replicates those from a number of other studies (e.g. Eskin, 1995; Rey Gex *et al.*, 1998), although some studies have not found actual suicide in a family member to be associated with suicidal phenomena in adolescents (e.g. Eskin, 1995; Marcenko *et al.*, 1999). Again, this probably reflects the relative rarity of suicide. Evidence from several

studies of people of all ages points to increased risk of suicide and of deliberate self-harm being associated with a family history of suicidal behaviour
(e.g. Roy, 2000; Statham *et al.*, 1998)

Exposure to suicidal behaviour in the family may have a modelling influence, such that family members may feel more comfortable with the idea of
suicide or be more likely to think of it at times of severe distress. The clustering of suicidal behaviour in families may also reflect a genetic risk for
specific psychiatric disorders. However, it appears to increase risk of suicidal
behaviour irrespective of specific disorders (Roy, 2000), suggesting that
there are genetic influences on personality characteristics, such as aggression
(Mann *et al.*, 1999), which may contribute to suicide risk. It is also possible
that suicidal behaviour by a family member might, in some circumstances,
deter other members of the family from engaging in suicidal behaviour. This
may depend on how the fact of suicide by a family member is dealt with, the
nature of the act, the relationship between the person who engaged in
suicidal behaviour and other family members, and the specific impact of the
event on individual family members.

Influence of the media

We did not investigate the possible association between suicidal phenomena
and exposure to suicidal behaviour in the media in our schools study. Also,
perhaps surprisingly, we have found only one community survey of adolescents in which this has been examined. A significant direct association with
suicide attempts (but not suicidal ideation) was found in an Australian study
for television viewing of suicides, surgery and funerals (Martin, 1996).
There is now substantial evidence that media reporting and portrayal of
suicidal behaviour can be a contributory factor in suicidal behaviour, especially in young people (Hawton and Williams, 2001; Pirkis and Blood,
2001; Schmidtke and Schaller, 2000). Associations have also been established between other behaviours and media portrayal in adolescence. For
example, Sargent and colleagues (2002) found a strong direct independent
association between adolescents seeing tobacco use in films and their trying
cigarettes. There is similarly good evidence that violent imagery in television, film and computer games has substantial short-term effects, increasing
the likelihood of aggressive or fearful behaviour in younger children, especially in boys, although the evidence is less consistent when older children
and teenagers are considered (Browne and Hamilton-Giachritsis, 2005).

The ways in which portrayal or reporting of suicide in the media may influence risk of suicidal behaviour, including self-harm, by others may be somewhat complex. Similar mechanisms may explain the increased risk of engaging in suicidal behaviour when an individual is exposed to deliberate self-harm and suicide among friends and family members. Some people have used an infection model to explain such influences (Gould and Davidson, 1988; Phillips 1980). Thus, transmission of the behaviour may depend on the virulence of the suicide model (e.g. the degree of esteem in which the model is held, the extent to which a person can identify with the person), the extent of exposure (e.g. repeated exposure having a greater influence), the susceptibility of the person who is exposed (e.g. mood, self-esteem) and protective factors (e.g. availability of other means of coping with feelings, availability of emotional supports). This model could also explain why outbreaks of self-harming behaviour may be more likely in institutional or relatively closed settings, such as schools and adolescent psychiatric inpatient units. This type of model cannot, however, explain fully the psychological mechanisms that are involved.

A further component in the process of contagious spread of suicidal behaviour is that of identification – that is, the tendency of individuals to imitate others with whom they feel they have a connection. Two types of identification have been distinguished: vertical, which is identification with celebrities and other high-status people (i.e. of higher status than the individidual), and horizontal, which is identification with people who share similar problems and/or personal characteristics with the individual (Stack, 1991). Vertical identification may explain why death by suicide of celebrities such as Marilyn Monroe and Japanese pop star Yukiko Okada (Takahashi, 1998) appear to have had such a profound influence on suicidal behaviour in the general population. Horizontal identification may be at the level of age or nationality and, perhaps more importantly, in terms of specific problems, such as relationship difficulties. This may explain why certain fictional television stories appear to have resulted in increases in self-harm and suicide (e.g. Hawton *et al.*, 1999c; Schmidtke and Häfner, 1988).

A further possible psychological process that may have additional relevance is that of projective identification, in which an individual may project certain qualities on to the person who has engaged in a suicidal act which may reflect their own characteristics or problems, such that the perceived boundary between that individual and the person who has engaged in the suicidal act becomes blurred. However, there is currently no evidence for or against this possibility.

The principles of social learning theory are also likely to be important, including the perceived outcomes or consequences of the suicidal behaviour. If these are perceived as positive in some way, such as through changing the behaviour of others, escape from problems or revenge, then this may influence the adoption of self-harm or suicide by an individual. Further influences may include restrictive thinking, with an excessive and possibly increasing focus by the individual on their problems and means of escaping from these, and rumination about and mental rehearsal of behaviour witnessed in others. In addition, exposure to suicidal behaviour in the media or by others may desensitise an individual to certain aspects of the behaviour, e.g. pain, and thus further reduce the threshold to engaging in suicidal behaviour. Finally, there may be specific modelling of a method of suicidal behaviour. This possibility is in keeping with the findings of studies of media portrayal and reporting of self-harm and suicide. Thus, the death of Yukiko Okada by jumping from a building was followed by a very marked increase in jumping as a method of suicide in young people in Japan (Takahashi, 1998); the death by jumping under a railway train of the 19-year-old hero of a German television series led to an increase in railway suicides in young people (Schmidtke and Häfner, 1988); and portrayal of a paracetamol overdose in the BBC television series *Casualty* was followed by a very marked increase in the use of paracetamol for overdose in viewers of the programme (Hawton *et al.*, 1999c).

Music

In spite of there often being anecdotal claims that certain types of popular music may be related to self-harm and suicidal acts by adolescents, there has been a dearth of investigations of this possible phenomenon. As long ago as 1975, heavy metal music was blamed for the deaths of two 14-year-old boys, who apparently were attempting to imitate a mock suicide by hanging performed on stage by Alice Cooper (Garner, 1975). Concerns have also been expressed about specific content of song lyrics with a pro-suicide flavour, although there is only limited research evidence that these have any specific impact on the behaviour of individuals.

Most of the attention to musical influences has been on heavy metal music. Arnett (1991) found that a liking for heavy metal music was associated with reckless behaviour among both male and female American high-school students. Male fans of heavy metal music reported more reckless driving, more sexual behaviour and more drug use than other adolescents, while female fans were more likely than other females to have engaged in shoplifting, vandalism, sexual behaviour and drug use; these girls also reported lower levels of self-esteem (Arnett, 1991).

In Australia, Martin and colleagues (1993) asked high-school students to complete a questionnaire about their musical preferences, risk-taking behaviours and other risk factors for suicidal behaviour. A preference for rock or heavy metal music was related to delinquency, risk-taking, drug and alcohol use, and family divorce or separation. This applied to both genders, but there was a strong gender bias in other findings. For example, only 26 per cent of girls preferred rock or heavy metal music, compared with 70.7 per cent of boys. Girls who preferred rock or heavy metal music were more likely to report suicidal thoughts, deliberate self-harm and depression than girls who listened to pop music (Martin *et al.*, 1993). Similar findings were reported for a study of a slightly older sample of American high-school students, who answered questions about their reasons for living, suicide factors and moods when listening to their favourite music (Scheel and Westfeld, 1999). Heavy metal fans indicated fewer reasons for living on a reasons for living inventory compared with subjects who listened to rock, rap, alternative or country music. Associations with suicidal ideas were found in both genders in this study (Scheel and Westfield, 1999). However, the association between suicidal ideas and heavy metal music was far more marked in girls. A similar finding emerged from the study of Martin and colleagues (1993) in Australia. It is possible that because a liking for heavy metal music is less common in girls, it may more often signal problems such as low self-esteem. Also, a liking for the misogynist portrayal of females in heavy metal music may contribute to or reinforce low self-esteem among female fans (Arnett, 1991).

In contrast with this possible conclusion, although Bjarnason and Thorlindsson (1994) found that listening to music and going to rock concerts were associated significantly with suicide attempts in both girls and boys in Iceland, in multivariate analysis controlling for a wide range of variables, listening to music, but not going to rock concerts, was found to have a significant association with suicide attempts in only boys.

Thus, preference for heavy metal music has been linked to suicidal behaviour, suicidal ideation and risk factors for suicidal behaviour in teenagers. This association appears to be stronger in females than in males. However, the cross-sectional nature of studies that have been mentioned makes it impossible to conclude that there is a causal influence between the music and suicidal ideation and self-harm. It is difficult to separate out the influence of the music from other risk factors, such as substance abuse, poor relationships with parents, alienation, low self-esteem and depression, all of which, as we have already discussed, are known to contribute to suicidal thinking and self-harm. More sophisticated investigations are required in order to elucidate the nature of the association between music and deliberate self-harm.

There is evidence that the context in which music occurs may have some relevance to its possible influence on suicidal phenomena. In a study in the USA, college students who watched a rock music video with a suicidal content subsequently wrote more scenarios with suicide-related themes in a projective story-telling task than those exposed to a rock music video without suicidal content. However, there was no difference between the groups of young people on measures of mood, attitudes and perceptions that might be related to suicidal behaviour (Rustad *et al.*, 2003). Thus, the suicidal content of music might have some influence on thinking related to suicide.

Summary and implications

In this chapter, we have described the factors that are associated with deliberate self-harm and suicidal thoughts by considering the results from our schools study as well as the findings from other studies reported in the international literature. In particular, we have focused upon associations with gender, ethnicity, psychosocial factors, mental health, bullying, substance use, smoking and certain family characteristics. We have also considered the effects of exposure to deliberate self-harm and suicide by friends and family members and in the media. Lastly, we have examined the limited evidence on the role, if any, of musical preference and exposure to certain types of music in risk of deliberate self-harm.

In our schools study, deliberate self-harm was nearly four times more frequent in females than in males. The results from research in a number of other countries suggest that this trend is internationally consistent. In other words, adolescent females are more likely than males to report suicide attempts and deliberate self-harm and to have thoughts of self-harm. This finding is also in keeping with studies that rely on data obtained from hospital admissions, in which the average rate of deliberate self-harm in adolescents is consistently higher in females.

In our schools study, we considered the prevalence of deliberate self-harm according to ethnic background separately for males and females. We found that although Asian females were significantly less likely to report self-harm than white females, there was no significant difference in rates of deliberate self-harm by ethnic group among the males in our sample. Our analysis of the international literature highlighted a general trend for suicidal phenomena to be more frequent in indigenous native populations. However, we also highlighted research that suggests it is important to bear in mind whether the population being studied is also a minority group geographically. In other words, it is important to look at whether members of the ethnic group live in an area in which they are in a minority, or whether they constitute a much larger proportion of the population in the area in which they live.

We also explored psychosocial and health characteristics. First, we looked at mental health and well-being and noted that levels of depression and anxiety in adolescents in our schools study were associated with deliberate self-harm in both males and females, but that the association was much stronger in females. We also found a link between impulsivity and deliberate self-harm among the females in our sample. Finally, we found that self-esteem was one of the factors associated most strongly with deliberate self-harm for both males and females.

In terms of substance use, we found that drug use, alcohol use and smoking were all associated with deliberate self-harm in our schools study. Drug use was one of the stronger predictors of deliberate self-harm for both the male and the female adolescents. The results of other studies support this finding and suggest that the association is stronger for hard drugs such as cocaine and heroin than for softer drugs such as cannabis. For both alcohol use and smoking, there was an increase in the risk of deliberate self-harm the more an individual drank or smoked in a typical week. However, the analyses suggested that the relationship between smoking and alcohol use and deliberate self-harm may not be direct but may be mediated by other factors.

We also focused on other personal characteristics and experiences of adolescents in our schools study. We found that having problems with keeping up with schoolwork was associated significantly with self-harm.

Peer relationships were also important: having difficulty keeping friends and having arguments with friends were significantly associated with increased prevalence of deliberate self-harm and thoughts of self-harm. Other research has suggested that although the negative aspects of peer relationships increase the likelihood of deliberate self-harm, positive aspects do not appear to act as a protective factor.

Adolescents in our schools study who said that they had been forced verbally or physically to engage in sexual activities against their will were at greater risk of deliberate self-harm than were their peers. There is also considerable evidence from other studies of adolescents for a strong and direct association between sexual abuse and suicidal phenomena. Similarly, physical abuse and bullying were associated with deliberate self-harm in our study.

We also highlighted the possible association between suicidal phenomena and sexual orientation. We found a significant association of deliberate self-harm with concerns about sexual orientation, although this did not appear to be a direct association, perhaps reflecting the relatively low rate of reporting of these concerns. This finding is in keeping with those reported by other researchers, who have found elevated rates of suicidal phenomena in homosexual and bisexual young people.

One factor that was associated particularly strongly with deliberate self-harm in our schools study was having a friend who had recently self-harmed. For both males and females, this was one of the strongest predictors of deliberate self-harm. This principally applied to self-cutting. Furthermore, self-harm by a family member was also a strong predictor of deliberate self-harm. It is possible that both experiences may have a modelling effect on adolescent behaviour.

Although we did not investigate the possible association between suicidal phenomena and exposure to suicidal behaviour in the media in our schools study, we felt it was important to draw attention to the fact that there is now substantial evidence that media reporting and portrayal of suicidal behaviour can be a contributory factor in suicidal behaviour, especially in young people. This issue is covered in greater depth in Chapter 8.

Finally, we have discussed the limited evidence regarding an association between musical preferences of adolescents, especially heavy metal music, and a possible increased risk of self-harm. The little research that has been conducted in this area suggests that this type of association may be stronger in girls than in boys.

Having highlighted the factors that appear to be associated with an increased likelihood of adolescents engaging in deliberate self-harm, or thinking about self-harm, in the next chapter we focus on the different sources of help and support that adolescents feel are available to them and, in particular, the kinds of coping strategy that adolescents use when they are experiencing problems.

CHAPTER 5

Adolescents' Help-seeking, Coping Strategies and Attitudes and Their Relevance to Deliberate Self-harm

Introduction

It is important to know what sources of help and support adolescents feel are available to them, but it is also crucial to know whether they use them. In this chapter, we consider help-seeking and how this differs between adolescents who self-harm and other adolescents. We also look at how attitudes to help-seeking may explain any such differences. It is also important to know what coping methods adolescents use, and how these differ between those who have and have not self-harmed as well as those who have had thoughts of self-harm but have not acted upon them. Identifying whether the coping strategies employed by adolescents who engage in deliberate self-harm or who have had thoughts of self-harm are different from those employed by other adolescents could inform the planning of interventions and enable them to be better targeted. Furthermore, identifying the people with whom adolescents feel able to talk provides valuable information on which people need to be prepared to support adolescents with problems. It may also pinpoint potential sources of help for adolescents that currently they are not utilising. Another relevant aspect of deliberate self-harm in adolescents concerns the attitudes of adolescents in general towards self-harmers and how this might vary between those who self-harm and those who do not. In this chapter, we explore all of these important aspects of deliberate self-harm in relation to the adolescents who took part in our schools study. We also relate the findings to those of other studies identified through our review of the international literature.

Help-seeking, communication and coping

It has been well documented that a substantial proportion of adolescents who deliberately self-harm or have thoughts of self-harm do not receive help (Choquet and Ledoux, 1994; Kann *et al.*, 2000). However, whether adolescents with such problems are able to recognise the extent of the difficulties they are facing is less clear. For example, a study of American adolescents found that only about half of the adolescents with thoughts of self-harm recognised that they needed help (Saunders *et al.*, 1994). In addition, young people can often be at a particular disadvantage not only in terms of recognising their own problems and needs but also in being able to communicate these problems and needs to others. For example, in her excellent book on self-harm and suicide in young people, Hill (1995) noted that many young people express despair through behaviour, not words, and end up isolated. She cited the example of a boy who did not have the vocabulary to describe his feelings and his situation and so injured himself with knives on a number of occasions following attacks of anxiety and despair. 'He had no choice, he reflected, between injuring himself and confiding in his parents. Without the insight or words to describe his tension and depression, he could not ask for help' (Hill, 1995: p.171). Similarly, both Rey Gex and colleagues (1998) in Switzerland and Wagman Borowsky and colleagues (1999) in the USA found that adolescents who did not talk about their problems were more likely to turn to deliberate self-harm.

Other studies have found that fewer adolescents who have had thoughts of self-harm said they would seek professional help compared with their peers who were not experiencing such problems but who were asked what they would do if they did have thoughts of self-harm (e.g. Carlton and Deane, 2000). Furthermore, several epidemiological studies have found that good communication with family members and feeling understood by them are associated with a lower prevalence of suicidal phenomena (e.g. Kandel *et al.*, 1991; Shaffer *et al.*, 1996). Wagman Borowsky and colleagues (1999) reported a similar association for discussing problems with family or friends. However, little attention has been paid to either the association between suicidal phenomena and communication with other potential helpers who can provide social support or what it is that influences whether or not adolescents choose to talk to someone and seek support.

Two dominant models can be identified within the social support literature: the main effect model (Ganster and Victor, 1988), which suggests that social support brings benefits, irrespective of the amount of stress encountered by the individual, and the buffer model (Cohen and Wills, 1985), which suggests that social support acts as a buffer against the negative effects of stress. Thus, different types of social support may benefit the individual. For example, emotional support, perhaps in the form of esteem-enhancing positive regard from others, may increase an individual's confidence in his or her ability to deal with challenges. On the other hand, informational support may help the individual to identify new strategies for resolving particular problems, and practical support may result in other resources being offered in order to help resolve problems.

However, although the theories and models suggest that social support may benefit the individual, the process of gaining social support means that the individual must enter a network of social relations. This may be very difficult for someone who has low self-esteem or high levels of depression and anxiety, all of which (as discussed in the previous chapter) increase the risk of deliberate self-harm. Social relationships by their very nature tend to demand a degree of reciprocity, which the individual with limited resources may not feel equipped to provide (Wainwright and Calnan, 2002).

In addition to lacking the ability to recognise or verbalise problems, it is possible that adolescents who engage in deliberate self-harm or who have thoughts of self-harm have poorer or inappropriate coping strategies compared with other adolescents. In this field, Lazarus and Folkman's (1984) transactional model has had a large impact on our understanding of the process of coping and suggests that the coping response is determined both by an individuals appraisal of the degree of threat posed and by the resources seen as being available to help him or her cope with the situation. So, the individual engages in an appraisal of the situation, which takes place in two stages: first the magnitude of the stressor is assessed, and second the individual assesses his or her perceived ability to cope with the stressor. Appraisal of a potential stressor can have three outcomes: it may be perceived as irrelevant, beneficial or potentially harmful. However, whether a stressor triggers a stress response will depend on the individual's appraisal of his or her ability to cope with the potential stressor. If an individual positively appraises his or her capacity to cope with a potential stressor, then this will greatly reduce the experience of stress (Wainwright and Calnan, 2002). This process of appraisal can be used to explain why some people cope or even thrive in circumstances that others would find unbearably stressful.

Researchers have distinguished between problem-focused and emotion-focused coping styles. The former involves using practical skills, especially interpersonal skills, to arrive at a practical solution to the problem. Emotion-focused coping involves controlling the emotional response to the stressor, for example by avoidance, denial or humour. Thus, an individual employing a problem-focused coping approach would attempt to actively alter the stressful situation in some way, perhaps by talking to someone about it, whilst a person employing an emotion-focused strategy would focus not on the cause of their stress but on their response to the stressful situation. The suggestion is that problem-focused strategies are more effective than emotion-focused strategies (e.g. Carver *et al.*, 1993). Identifying whether the coping strategies employed by adolescents who engage in deliberate self-harm or who have thoughts of self-harm differ from those employed by other adolescents would contribute to our knowledge of what types of intervention might be most effective with respect to emotion-focused versus problem-focused strategies.

In our schools study we have investigated these processes in relation to adolescents with thoughts of self-harm or who carry out acts of deliberate self-harm in order to find out whether adolescents receive help and, if not, whether this is because they do not recognise that they need help (Evans *et al.*, 2005b). Furthermore, we asked the adolescents about the people with whom they felt able to talk. This was in order to provide us with potentially valuable information about the people that need to be prepared to support adolescents with problems and may pinpoint potential sources of help for adolescents that are currently not being utilised.

Recognition of problems and the need for help

Overall, 27.2 per cent of the sample of adolescents in our schools study identified themselves as having had recent serious personal, emotional, behavioural or mental health problems. In males, such problems were reported by 62.1 per cent with an episode of deliberate self-harm in the previous year, 49.0 per cent with thoughts of self-harm and 15.3 per cent of the remainder. There was a similar pattern in females, these types of problems being reported by, respectively, 78.3 per cent of those with an episode of deliberate self-harm, 48.4 per cent of those with thoughts of self-harm and 20.8 per cent of the remainder (Table 5.1).

Among adolescents who identified themselves as having serious problems, fewer of those with a deliberate self-harm episode in the previous year or recent thoughts of self-harm had felt the need for help compared with those without a deliberate self-harm episode or those who had had thoughts of deliberate self-harm. This applied to both genders (Table 5.1). By contrast, the proportion of adolescents who reported that they had felt the need for help but did not try to get any was greatest in those with a deliberate self-harm episode and lowest in those with neither deliberate self-harm nor thoughts of self-harm. There was little difference in the proportions of adolescents with problems in the three groups who had felt the need for help and asked for it, but females with deliberate self-harm were significantly more likely to report this than their peers. Thus, although more adolescents with problems who had had a deliberate self-harm episode felt the need to get help, fewer of them had actually done so.

Coping strategies employed by adolescents

In our schools study, adolescents who reported that they had engaged in deliberate self-harm in the past year were asked whether they had tried to get help beforehand and whether they had received help for their most recent self-harm episode. Less than half (46.7%) of the adolescents who had self-harmed reported that they had tried to get help beforehand. Just over half (55.0%) of the adolescents had received help after the last deliberate self-harm episode.

We asked all the adolescents to choose from a list of eight coping strategies and indicate how frequently (never/sometimes/often) they employed each approach listed when they were worried or upset (Figure 5.1). Overall, the most frequently endorsed response was that they tried to sort things out at least sometimes. Other common coping strategies included getting angry and talking to someone. The least frequently chosen method for coping when worried or upset was having an alcoholic drink, although this option was endorsed by a substantial proportion (40%) of the adolescents.

We divided the adolescents into three groups:

- those who reported having engaged in deliberate self-harm
- those who reported having had thoughts of self-harm
- those who reported neither self-harm nor thoughts of self-harm.

Table 5.1 Pupils who identified themselves as having serious personal, emotional, behavioural or mental health problems: recognition of need for help and whether help was sought.

	Deliberate self-harm n(%)	*Thoughts of self-harm n(%)*	*No self-harm or thoughts of self-harm n(%)*	*Chi squared for trend* P
Serious problems				
Males	59/95 (62.1)	120/245 (49.0)	374/2445 (15.3)	<0.0005
Females	227/290 (78.3)	281/580 (48.4)	347/1669 (20.8)	<0.0005
Of those with serious problems				
Did not feel the need for help				
Males	16/59 (27.1)	46/120 (38.3)	175/374 (46.8)	<0.003
Females	69/227 (30.4)	105/281 (37.4)	171/347 (49.3)	<0.0005
Felt the need for help but did not try to get any				
Males	31/59 (52.5)	54/120 (45.0)	123/374 (32.9)	<0.001
Females	96/227 (42.3)	113/281 (40.2)	100/347 (28.8)	<0.001
Felt the need for help and asked for it				
Males	12/59 (20.3)	20/120 (16.7)	76/374 (20.3)	no trend
Females	62/227 (27.3)	63/281 (22.4)	76/347 (21.9)	<0.0005

Adapted from Evans *et al.* (2005b), with permission.

It was clear that the coping strategies employed differed between the three groups for both males and females (Figure 5.2).

Overall, the most notable difference between the three groups was having an alcoholic drink when worried or upset, which was reported by far more of those with a history of deliberate self-harm or thoughts of self-harm. Adolescents with a history of deliberate self-harm were more likely than other adolescents to report staying in their rooms. Females who had self-harmed were more likely to report getting angry than other females (Figure 5.2b). More males and females who had engaged in deliberate self-harm appeared to use these kinds of emotion-focused behaviours when responding to a stressful situation rather than actively dealing with the cause of the stress (Figure 5.2). Although adolescents without any history of self-harm or thoughts of self-harm were more likely than others to report employing problem-focused approaches, such as trying to sort things out and talking to someone, they were also more likely to employ the emotion-focused strategy of trying not to think about what it was that was worrying them (Figure 5.1)

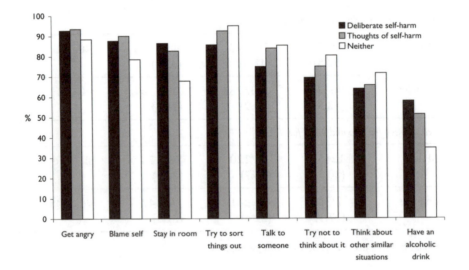

Figure 5.1 Coping strategies employed by adolescents in our schools study when faced with stressful situations according to history of deliberate self-harm, thoughts of self-harm or neither. Adapted from Evans et al. (2005b), with permission.

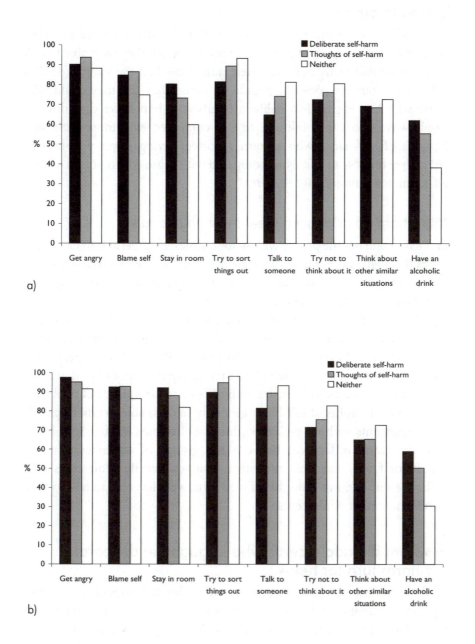

Figure 5.2 Coping strategies employed by adolescents in our schools study when faced with stressful situations, according to history of deliberate self-harm, thoughts of self-harm or neither. (a) Males; (b) females. Adapted from Evans et al. (2005b), with permission.

Talking to others

Almost all the adolescents in our schools study (95.4%) reported that they had at least one category of person to whom they felt they were able to talk about things that really bothered them; just under half the sample (45.7%) had at least four categories of people to whom they felt they could talk. Those who had engaged in deliberate self-harm had fewer categories of people with whom they felt able to talk compared with those with only thoughts of self-harm, who in turn reported having fewer people with whom they felt able to talk when compared with those who reported neither self-harm nor thoughts of self-harm.

With whom do adolescents feel most able to talk?

It is vital to find out the people with whom adolescents feel able to talk about things that really bother them if we are going to be able to effectively target advice and education regarding how best to help people who are struggling with thoughts or acts of deliberate self-harm.

Almost 85 per cent of the adolescents in our schools study said that they felt that they were able to talk to a friend about things that really bothered them. This was followed in frequency by mothers (67%). Only 20 per cent of adolescents felt that they could talk to their teachers about things that really bothered them. Males and females with a history of an episode of deliberate self-harm or thoughts of self-harm generally felt less able to talk to people than adolescents without such thoughts or behaviours (Figure 5.3). There were significant differences between the groups of adolescents in this respect for family members and other relatives. Female adolescents with deliberate self-harm or thoughts of self-harm were less able to talk to their friends than other adolescents.

To whom did adolescents who engaged in deliberate self-harm turn for help?

Of those adolescents in our schools study who had sought help before engaging in deliberate self-harm, females (49.8%) were more likely than males (36.7%) to have tried to get help from at least one source beforehand. In general, the most common potential source of help to whom the adolescents had turned was a friend (41.0%) (Figure 5.4). Females (43.8%) were more likely than males (31.9%) to have tried to get help from a friend.

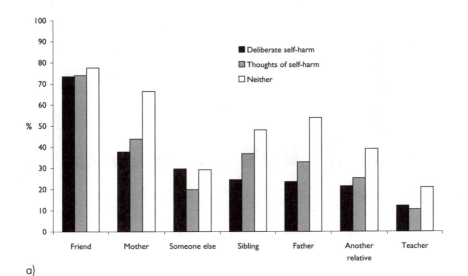

a)

b)

Figure 5.3 People with whom adolescents in our schools study felt that they could talk about problems, according to history of deliberate self-harm, thoughts of self-harm or neither. (a) Males; (b) females. Adapted from Evans et al. (2005b), with permission.

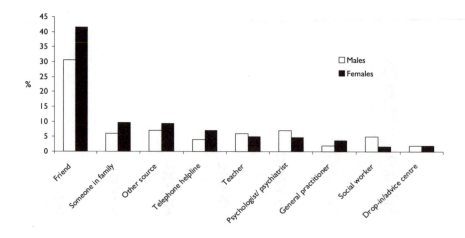

Figure 5.4 Sources of help approached by adolescents in our schools study engaging in deliberate self-harm, by gender. From Evans et al. *(2005b), with permission.*

Adolescents who had engaged in deliberate self-harm were asked to indicate from a list who (if anyone) knew about what they did on the last occasion that they had harmed themselves. In almost 80 per cent of cases, at least one person knew about the adolescent's episode of deliberate self-harm. Friends were most likely to know (72.4%), followed by mothers (26%) and siblings (24%). This pattern was the same for both genders.

What stopped adolescents from seeking help?

Overall, 53 per cent of the adolescents in our schools study who had engaged in deliberate self-harm said that they had not tried to seek help beforehand. They were asked to explain in their own words why they had not sought help. A small number of adolescents said that this was because they had wanted to die. However, by far the most common answers given to the question were that they had not needed or wanted any help:

Because I didn't want help.

I didn't need it. I could get through on my own and I did better than if anyone had helped me.

I'm not an attention seeker. I don't want or need help from anyone especially not in that state of mind.

Other adolescents explained that they thought that their problem was not serious enough for them to seek help:

I did not feel it was serious enough for help.

I didn't feel it was important enough.

My problems seem small compared to the world problems and I don't want to be ungrateful for what I have.

Didn't feel my problems were important enough.

Other adolescents acknowledged that they had problems but felt that they should deal with them themselves:

Because it was my problem to face by myself.

Because it was my problem and I had to deal with it in my own way.

Because I don't talk about my problems because they are *MY* problems.

There was also often a certain element of shame mixed with fear about how others might react. As a result, a large number of adolescents were concerned about other people knowing what they were doing:

I didn't want to tell anyone, because I was embarrassed.

I was ashamed.

I didn't want people to worry about me and I didn't like people to think of me as depressing.

Linked to this was the notion that other people would not understand why the adolescents engaged in this kind of behaviour. Some adolescents were particularly worried that their behaviour would be seen as attention-seeking:

Because people might think I was a stupid little girl who just wanted attention. I didn't think anyone could help me then.

> Because if I said to anyone, look I'm fed up of life so I'm going to take an overdose, and they would just say I've got no sympathy for you – carry on.

> I was frightened people would think I was just trying to get sympathy and attention, which I wasn't.

> Because I felt as though no one would understand me and that they would think I was being a stupid attention seeker or it was just my hormones etc. I felt no one could see exactly why I was doing it.

Sadly, a small number of adolescents mentioned that they felt that no one would be able to help them or would want to help:

> I didn't feel anyone could help me any more.

> I didn't think that anyone would actually want to listen. Why would anybody want to listen to me when there was nothing specifically wrong with me? I just felt depressed.

> Because I didn't feel as though anyone cared about me enough to care if I tried to kill myself.

Did adolescents who had thoughts of self-harm seek help?

Adolescents from our schools study who reported thoughts of self-harm but had not actually engaged in deliberate self-harm in the past year were asked whether they had talked to or tried to get help from certain sources. Sixty per cent of adolescents in this category had talked to or tried to get help from at least one source, with significantly more females (63.6%) than males (50.4%) having done so. Help was most often sought from friends (49.9%); the second but much less frequently used source of help was family members (18.3%). Males were more likely than females to have talked to or tried to get help from a psychologist or psychiatrist.

Attitudes towards young people who engage in deliberate self-harm

Self-harming behaviour often arouses intense negative reactions in others, including clinicians and the general public (Gratz, 2003). We were very interested in finding out about how the adolescents in our schools study viewed young people who engaged in deliberate self-harm. In order to do this, we asked all the adolescents who completed our questionnaire about their attitudes towards young people who harmed themselves. They were asked to indicate whether they agreed with five statements about young people who engaged in deliberate self-harm.

We compared the responses from adolescents who had engaged in self-harm with those who had had thoughts of self-harm and those who had not engaged in either behaviour (Table 5.2). We found that similar percentages from the three groups considered that most young people who harmed themselves were lonely and depressed. Similarly, the statement that most young people who harmed themselves could have been prevented from

Table 5.2 Responses of adolescents in our schools study to statements about attitudes towards people who harm themselves (percentages in agreement), according to whether in the previous year they had self-harmed, had thoughts of self-harm or neither

	Deliberate self-harm (%)	Thoughts of self-harm (%)	Neither (%)
Most young people who harm themselves are lonely and depressed	61.5	63.4	62.6
Most young people who harm themselves do it on the spur of the moment	32.4	21.1	19.4
Most young people who harm themselves are feeling suicidal	38.1	45.4	35.6
Most young people who harm themselves are trying to get attention	24.3	31.2	36.5
Most young people who harm themselves could have been prevented from doing so	51.3	57.8	55.0

doing so provoked little difference in opinion between the three groups, with slightly fewer of the respondents who had engaged in deliberate self-harm agreeing with the statement compared with the other two groups. Whether deliberate self-harm was an impulsive act was an area in which there were differences in opinion between the three groups. Almost a third (32.4%) of those respondents who had engaged in deliberate self-harm agreed that young people who harmed themselves did so on the spur of the moment, but only a fifth of those who had had thoughts of self-harm (21.1%) and those who had not engaged in either behaviour (19.4%) agreed with the statement. Similarly, those who had engaged in deliberate self-harm were more likely to express agreement with the statement that most young people who self-harm are feeling suicidal, while those who had not self-harmed or had thoughts of self-harm were least likely to agree with this statement.

In Chapter 3, we explored the motivation behind acts of deliberate self-harm and showed that the adolescents in our study were unlikely to explain their behaviour in terms of seeking attention. Although this result has also been found elsewhere (e.g. Favazza and Conterio, 1989; Hawton *et al.*, 1982a), it is important to emphasise it in order to counter the commonly held belief that people who carry out acts of deliberate self-harm use this behaviour as a means of seeking attention. The attitudes expressed by respondents in each of the three groups differed in that those who had engaged in deliberate self-harm were least likely to endorse the statement (24.3%), while those who had neither engaged in self-harm nor had thoughts of self-harm were the most likely to endorse this statement (36.5%). There were, therefore, some differences in terms of attitudes expressed in response to the five statements about young people who harm themselves, with the most notable differences concerning the impulsive nature of the act of deliberate self-harm and the notion that those who engage in deliberate self-harm are seeking attention.

Attitudes towards contacting helping agencies

Pupils in our schools study were asked to comment on helping agencies and how such agencies could best help other people of their age who were experiencing problems. A common theme to emerge from the responses to this question concerned the stigma that adolescents felt surrounded the issue of 'asking for help'. Several adolescents said they thought that young people may feel embarrassed about asking someone for help or may lack the confidence to actively seek help for fear that others will make fun of them:

> I don't know, but people might get embarrassed going to them and people might take the mickey out of them so that is why people don't always go to them.

> Most young people don't have enough confidence to call the helplines.

> Make it more appealing to everyone so people don't feel scared of asking for help.

Many adolescents expressed the view that young people needed to be made more aware of the crisis and helpline services that exist. This suggests that the advertising of such services needs to be better targeted, not only to improve awareness of the existence of the services but also to increase awareness of what the services offer. It also appeared that many of the adolescents were not aware that agencies could help with all kinds of problems, no matter how big or small:

> Make themselves more known.

> Publicity should be a major issue.

> In their adverts, they just seem to be helping those with huge problems, so they could show that they help those with small problems as people don't think that their problems are significant.

Although the adolescents often appeared to recognise the importance of having someone to turn to who would listen to their problems, they also often wanted helping agencies to offer advice and solutions to their problems. In addition, the need for people who work in helping agencies to be able to empathise with young people was emphasised. One suggestion that cropped up regularly was that agencies should recruit younger people as volunteers, who would then be more able to understand the problems of adolescents:

> To sit and listen to them, try to give advice that they could use, don't judge them.

> By listening to them and looking at the problems from a young person's view but with adult experience so that they can give good advice.

> By having people who have been through it themselves and have young people on the phone so that the caller can relate to them.

> We would need to talk to youngish people – 17–24 – that could relate to our problems and understand us and we may be able to trust them completely.

> They should have younger members so that youngsters like us can talk to them as young members have the right attitude to help.

Finally, a large number of the adolescents thought that having helping agencies visit their schools on a regular basis would be a good idea so that pupils would have the opportunity to talk to someone:

> Come to schools and ask children out of class (interview them) if they have any problems they wish to discuss.

> Come into schools on a regular basis and talk to every child.

> Visit a lot more schools so that young people know what it was all about.

Summary and implications

The majority of adolescents in our schools study who had engaged in deliberate self-harm and about half of those who had experienced thoughts of self-harm indicated that they felt that they had had recent serious personal, emotional, behavioural or mental health problems. In some cases, thoughts of self-harm might reflect a stage of adolescence in which the concept of an individual's own mortality is developing rather than being a sign that something is seriously wrong, in which case it is perhaps not so surprising that many adolescents who have thoughts of self-harm do not think they have serious problems. In other cases, however, thoughts of self-harm will reflect major distress and may lead to actual self-harm or suicidal acts.

What is more worrying is the finding that a quarter of adolescents who reported having actually engaged in deliberate self-harm did not consider that they had a serious problem. This is in keeping with Saunders and colleagues' (1994) finding that only about half of American adolescents with thoughts of deliberate self-harm recognised that they needed help. This suggests that adolescents may need help in order to recognise that they have problems, to identify what those problems are, and to assess their severity.

Compared with their peers, adolescents in our schools study who had carried out acts of deliberate self-harm and those with thoughts of self-harm mentioned fewer categories of people with whom they felt able to talk about things that really bothered them. This means that their social support resources were poorer than those of other adolescents. For most of those adolescents with a history of a recent deliberate self-harm episode, at least one person knew about it, but worryingly more than 20 per cent reported that no one knew. Similarly, of those adolescents who reported having experienced thoughts of self-harm, 40 per cent had not talked to or tried to get help from anyone. Further research is needed to establish whether it is the lack of support that results in suicidal phenomena or, conversely, whether there is a tendency for adolescents who are experiencing problems to isolate themselves from the support that could be offered by their social network. Alternatively, it is possible that adolescents with problems have fewer people to whom they can turn because their problems have driven their sources of support away. This is an issue that would need to be investigated longitudinally in order to see whether a causal relationship can be established.

In terms of to whom specifically adolescents reported that they felt they could talk, it is not surprising that the vast majority in our study felt able to talk to their friends about things that really bothered them. Furthermore, if help was sought before a deliberate self-harm episode, then it was most commonly sought from friends. Friends were also most likely to know about a deliberate self-harm episode and to try to provide help after the episode. Similarly, adolescents with thoughts of self-harm were most likely to seek help from their peers. These findings suggest that adolescents need to be provided with education and advice on how best to help friends with problems, including deliberate self-harm and thoughts of self-harm. This may seem a large burden to place on adolescents, but clearly if they are the main potential source of support for troubled peers then they need help in managing this important role. This could be done in the context of mental health education programmes in schools (see Chapter 6). Such programmes should include advice on when an adolescent needs to seek help for a peer from adults, even if this might involve breaching confidentiality in order to best help a friend and perhaps prevent a suicidal act.

Teachers were viewed relatively rarely as a source of help by adolescents. It may be that pupils are afraid that if they confide in a teacher, then others in the school setting will find out about their behaviour or problems. Further research is therefore required to explore why teachers are not being utilised as a source of help and support by distressed pupils. Given that teachers are likely to be the only adults other than parents or guardians with whom the adolescents will have regular contact, it is likely that teachers would also benefit from education and advice on how best to help pupils who engage in deliberate self-harm or who have thoughts of self-harm. Teachers would certainly need considerable support from other agencies if they are to adopt this kind of supportive role.

The adolescents in our study who had engaged in deliberate self-harm or who had thoughts of self-harm indicated that they tended to use emotion-focused coping strategies, such as having an alcoholic drink or getting angry, when faced with problems. In contrast, adolescents without thoughts of self-harm or self-harm behaviours more often said that they employed strategies that focused actively on their problem, such as talking to someone or trying to sort things out. Although this does not necessarily mean that emotion-focused coping is always detrimental and that problem-focused coping is more effective, the difference we found between the subgroups of adolescents in our schools study is in keeping with findings from other studies that indicate that adolescents with deliberate self-harm are less able to solve problems effectively (Kingsbury *et al.*, 1999; Rotheram-Borus *et al.*, 1990) and are more likely to engage in emotion-focused coping, whereby they focus on their emotional response to the stressor rather than dealing with the root cause of the stressor. As a result, these adolescents may be less able to cope effectively with the stressors in their lives and are, therefore, at greater risk of repeat episodes of deliberate self-harm, which in some cases will lead to completed suicide.

Nearly two-thirds of the total sample of adolescents in our schools study, including those with a history of deliberate self-harm and those with thoughts of self-harm, considered adolescents who had engaged in deliberate self-harm to be lonely and depressed. However, more of the adolescents who had self-harmed considered the act to be often impulsive and to say that most self-harmers are feeling suicidal. It is problable that the appraisal of self-harmers by those who have engaged in deliberate self-harm is likely to be more realistic.

In this chapter, we have explored the different help-seeking behaviours that distinguish adolescents who have carried out acts of deliberate self-harm or who have experienced thoughts of self-harm from adolescents who have experienced neither. In particular, we have explored the adolescents' coping strategies and their attitudes towards seeking help. Adolescents who have engaged in deliberate self-harm or who have experienced thoughts of self-harm are more likely to employ coping strategies that avoid the stressor and concentrate on the emotional response to the stressor. They are also likely to have fewer sources of social support to turn to when they are feeling worried or upset. Finally, they appear to view self-harmers and the act of self-harm somewhat differently to other adolescents. In Part 2, we discuss the implications of the findings from Part 1 for educators, schools, teachers, clinicians and crisis agencies.

Part 2

Prevention and Treatment of Deliberate Self-harm in Adolescents

CHAPTER 6

Schools and Deliberate Self-harm

Introduction

In the first part of this book, we focused on providing the reader with information concerning what is known about deliberate self-harm in adolescents. This information has been obtained both from our thorough review of the international literature and from our large schools study.

One of the key aims of our schools study was to establish the prevalence of deliberate self-harm and thoughts of self-harm in a large representative sample of adolescents in England. We presented our main findings in Part 1 of this book and have shown that the majority of cases of deliberate self-harm by adolescents do not result in presentation to hospital. Other research in England has shown that some young people who die by suicide have a history of previously undetected deliberate self-harm (Hawton *et al.*, 1999a) and that this is also the case in some young people who subsequently present to hospitals because of a further episode of deliberate self-harm (Hawton *et al.*, 1996).

In our schools study almost 7 per cent of adolescents reported engaging in deliberate self-harm in the past year. Similar surveys from the USA, Australia and other countries in Europe also suggest that this behaviour is common, with prevalence figures ranging from approximately 4 per cent to 10 per cent of adolescents reporting acts of deliberate self-harm in the year before being questioned. Furthermore, a sizeable proportion of adolescents think about but do not carry out acts of self-harm. In our schools study, 15 per cent of the sample had thought about deliberate self-harm in the previous year but had not engaged in the act. We have also shown that a large proportion of the adolescents who reported deliberate self-harm had not tried to seek help beforehand. Some said they had not sought help because they did not think that their problems were serious enough, while others felt that they really ought to deal with their problems themselves rather than turn to someone else. Perhaps of most concern was the fear about how others would react: many young people in our sample reported feeling embarrassed or ashamed of what they were planning to do or had done. Still more felt that other people would not understand why they were planning to harm themselves.

We know that a large proportion of those adolescents who engage in deliberate self-harm do so impulsively; for example, in our schools study, 50 per cent of those who cut themselves and 36 per cent of those who took overdoses said that they had thought about harming themselves for less than an hour beforehand. We also know that the vast majority of deliberate self-harm does not come to the attention of the medical profession: in our study, only 12.6 per cent of cases of deliberate self-harm had resulted in presentation to hospital. Thus, the combination of the impulsive nature of self-harming behaviour and the reluctance of adolescents to seek help other than from their friends means that there is often little time for intervention before the act once an adolescent has started to think about it.

In this chapter, we focus on schools. In particular, we look at school-based prevention strategies, detection of young people at risk and dealing with the aftermath of deliberate self-harm and suicide.

Why base prevention strategies in schools?

Wyn and colleagues (2000) highlight the fact that schools are only one of the places where the environment can affect young people's well-being. They state that although schools provide an attractive setting for prevention programmes, it would be simplistic to ignore the role of other areas of life in which young people's mental health and well-being are shaped. In contrast, Davis and Sandovel (1991) argue that the prevalence of suicidal behaviour among youths is such that every school and community should be prepared to deal with it.

There are sound reasons to consider schools as a suitable setting for prevention strategies. For example, our review of the international literature demonstrated a likely association between suicidal phenomena and many school-related variables, such as poor academic performance, poor school attendance and having a negative attitude towards school and schoolwork.

In addition, Patton and colleagues (2000) point out that schools are arguably the only point of almost universal access to young people at a time during which emotional problems and behaviours with long-lasting harmful effects on health commonly emerge. Klingman and Hochdorf (1993) suggest that schools are considered the best community location for primary prevention because the goal of many prevention programmes is compatible with the very goals of the educational process, namely optimising the students' adjustment and improving their quality of life.

A further point has been raised by American writers who have noted that there has been increasing concern with legal issues surrounding the responsibility and liability of the school with regard to teenage suicide. Miller and DuPaul (1996: p.221) noted that in the USA school districts 'can and have been sued for inadequate suicide prevention programmes'. On the other hand, they noted that legal issues are also a barrier for implementing suicide-prevention programmes because schools can find themselves in a 'no-win' situation where they can be legally accountable for not having prevention programmes in place and yet also may be criticised for offering such programmes (Davis *et al.*, 1988). Several cases have been brought against US schools claiming that school personnel had deficient training in suicide prevention (Poland, 1995).

Nevertheless, Kalafat and Elias (1995) argue that since children and adolescents spend much of their time in school, school-based programmes have been and are likely to remain the centrepiece of suicide prevention efforts. Shaffer and Gould (2000) expand this point and highlight three reasons why a school-based approach is appealing:

- Deliberate self-harm and thoughts of self-harm are common during the school years.

- Adolescents are gathered conveniently in schools, so that evaluations can be carried out or interventions provided in a cost-effective manner.

- Schools are a good place for treatment because teenagers attend school-based clinics more regularly than they do hospital clinics.

Another important reason for focusing on the school setting is that the majority of suicidal youths come to the attention of their peers rather than adults. These peer confidants may play a pivotal role in the prevention of youth suicide if they take responsible action on behalf of their troubled peers

(Kalafat and Elias, 1994). Thus school prevention programmes have a double role to play: to raise awareness of the sources of help that are available to young people who are engaging in self-harm and to better support, prepare and equip young people who may be the first port of call for a friend when he or she is thinking of or has already carried out an act of deliberate self-harm. School prevention programmes may play a vital role in teaching adolescents about when it is appropriate to break a friend's confidence and to whom they can turn for help themselves.

What approaches have been used in schools?

School-based prevention programmes can be considered in three categories:

- *Primary prevention,* where the aim is to modify factors that might predispose individuals to suicidal phenomena, e.g. changing attitudes or improving coping skills.

- *Secondary prevention,* which is targeted at individuals who have been identified as at risk but who have not yet made a suicide attempt.

- *Tertiary prevention,* which involves providing help for individuals who have made a suicide attempt. It can also include endeavouring to limit the impact of suicidal behaviour on others, such as peers and family members.

At each of these prevention levels, various agencies may be involved, for example schools, families, mental health professionals and helping organisations such as Samaritans and other telephone and crisis services.

Primary prevention

Suicide-awareness programmes

The most common approach to the primary prevention of adolescent suicide involves curriculum-based prevention or education programmes. Garland and colleagues (1989) conducted a national survey of suicide-prevention programmes in the USA and found that many adopted a universal strategy. In other words, the programmes were directed to all pupils, regardless of individual susceptibility, experience or vulnerability. They noted that the programmes tended to be based on two key assumptions:

- Suicide is a consequence of stress: because stress may be experienced by anyone, it can be argued that everyone is a potential suicide risk.

- Teenagers turn to other teenagers when in distress or in need of emotional support. The role of friends and peers in the early recognition of suicidal behaviour and prevention of suicide cannot be overemphasised (Shafi *et al.*, 1985).

As an approach to suicide prevention, these types of programme have received a lot of attention (Fox and Hawton, 2004). Many of these programmes aim to increase awareness of suicidal behaviour, with the goals of encouraging pupils to disclose their feelings and preparing adolescents to identify at-risk peers and training them to take 'responsible action' (Kalafat and Elias, 1994). Linked to this point, Kalafat and Elias (1995) highlight the fact that misconceptions about suicide have been associated with a failure to respond actively to suicidal peers. Thus, the idea is that the more that adolescents know about suicide warning signs and sources of help, the more likely they will be to ask for help for themselves or to encourage their peers to seek help.

Many programmes use some form of trigger to introduce the students to the topic of suicide. This may take the form of a vignette or a video (Hazell and King, 1996). Unfortunately, due to the tendency to choose attractive actors and to dramatise the action by showing explicit details of the suicide act, and by trivialising the precipitants to the suicide, such 'educational' videos often share most of the unwanted characteristics of news and fictional broadcasts of suicide that are thought to encourage imitation (see Chapter 8 for a discussion of media influences). Furthermore, Garland and colleagues (1989) raised the objection that programmes often minimise the contribution that psychiatric disorder makes to the problem of suicide and suicide behaviours. Hazell and King (1996) suggest that this is almost certainly a deliberate strategy to increase the acceptability of the programmes. This is supported by the findings of Garland and colleagues (1989), who reported that several programme directors indicated that they deliberately avoided a mental illness orientation in their programmes in favour of the stress model, because they assumed that emphasising the links between psychiatric illness and suicide would discourage disclosure of suicide intent by affected teenagers.

A typical school-based education programme aiming to increase awareness of the problem of suicide would review the epidemiology of adolescent suicide and then provide a description of warning signs that would encourage and help staff and students to identify others at risk. It would also aim to counteract permissive and positive attitudes about suicide (Fox and Hawton, 2004; Shaffer and Gould, 2000). However, Shaffer and Gould (2000) note that there is, as yet, no evidence that these excellent goals can be met by these programmes. Indeed, there is conflict in the published literature as to the effectiveness of such programmes, with some researchers warning that they may actually have a negative impact on the mental health of adolescents by increasing the acceptability of suicide (Shaffer et al., 1990). For example, some studies have found that the programmes resulted in an improvement in knowledge (Kalafat and Elias, 1994; Silbert and Berry, 1991) or attitudes (Kalafat and Gigliano, 1996), while other studies have reported either no benefits (e.g. Shaffer et al., 1990) or unfavourable effects (Overholser et al., 1989; Shaffer et al., 1991).

Concerns about the potentially harmful nature of suicide-awareness programmes that have been directed at students have led to demands for a focus on the problems facing adolescents rather than on youth suicide in particular (Beautrais et al., 1997). The Guidelines for Schools document compiled by Beautrais and colleagues presents a strong case for incorporating suicide-prevention messages within the context of positive mental health promotion programmes. The key considerations underlying this decision have been, first, the fear that suicide-awareness programmes for students may encourage them to view suicide as a legitimate response to their stress. Second, research has shown that a large proportion of young people dying by suicide or making suicide attempts will have had a recognisable psychiatric disorder before the suicide attempt (e.g. Beautrais et al., 1996; Burgess et al., 1998; Hawton et al., 1999a; Kerfoot et al., 1996; Shaffer et al., 1996). At present, there is insufficient evidence to either support or not support curriculum-based suicide-awareness programmes in schools (Gould et al., 2003). As a result, interest has moved towards an alternative approach to prevention that focuses instead on skills training for staff and/or pupils.

Skills training programmes

In contrast to raising awareness about suicidal behaviour, skills training programmes focus on targeting ways of addressing the problems that lead to thoughts of self-harm. This emphasis is on helping young people to acquire alternative methods of problem-solving, coping and cognitive skills and to recognise existing sources of help.

An example of such a programme is described by Klingman and Hochdorf (1993), who reported on a skills training programme they designed to improve adolescents' ability to cope with distress and to enhance their awareness of and response to peers in distress. Tools employed to teach the skills were selected vignettes used to aid role-playing improvisations, newspaper clips, handouts, written exercises and group discussion. Their intervention led to an improved awareness of coping responses and a lessened intent to commit suicide in boys. However, as pointed out by Shaffer and Gould (2000), further research is needed to see whether these changes in attitude are translated into actual changes in behaviour.

Mental health awareness programmes

Rather than focusing explicitly on deliberate self-harm and suicide, a third approach is to focus more generally on improving adolescents' awareness of mental health issues. There is increasing awareness of mental health problems in young people, with evidence that rates of depression in adolescents have risen over the past few decades (Fombonne, 1995; Klerman, 1988; Volkmar, 1996). In some cases, depression can lead to suicidal thoughts or actual acts of deliberate self-harm. Indeed, as discussed earlier, many adolescents who engage in acts of deliberate self-harm and present to hospital are suffering from psychiatric disorders, especially depression and anxiety (Burgess et al., 1998; Kerfoot et al., 1996). In our review of the international literature on school-based and community studies, we found that deliberate self-harm was associated strongly with psychiatric disorders, in particular depression and anxiety. Similarly, in our schools study, levels of depression and anxiety were significantly higher in those adolescents with a recent history of deliberate self-harm.

Although life events and difficulties will contribute to the mental health problems of adolescents, there is evidence to show that specific characteristics of adolescents may make them more vulnerable to the effects of stress. One factor is their level of problem-solving skills. Poor problem-solving ability has been linked to both depression (Adams and Adams, 1991, 1996; Sacco and Graves, 1984; Sadowski and Kelly, 1993) and suicidal behaviour (Kingsbury et al., 1999; Speckens and Hawton, 2005) in clinical and community samples of adolescents. Another important, although less studied, vulnerability factor is self-esteem, i.e. how individuals regard and value themselves. Adolescents with a history of deliberate self-harm in our schools study had lower self-esteem than other adolescents.

In addition to the characteristics that may make adolescents more vulnerable to the effects of stress, an important aspect of prevention of psychiatric problems and deliberate self-harm in adolescents is the extent to which they feel able to seek help. As we have noted already, young people see their peers as an important source of support. Indeed, Evans and colleagues (1996) found that adolescents rated having close friends as one of the most important sources of help when feeling suicidal or in a crisis. In addition, Hennig and colleagues (1998) found that 50 per cent of adolescents said that when they were in a crisis they were more likely to turn to a friend than a parent or counsellor. The responses of adolescents in our schools study indicate that many had found seeking help difficult and that they were often poorly informed about voluntary agencies and the kind of help that they can provide. Furthermore, even though adolescents see their peers as an important source of support, there are important questions concerning the extent to which they are able to (i) recognise when friends are having difficulties, (ii) provide help, either themselves or through involving other people, and (iii) know when it is both important and acceptable to break confidences in order to get help for a friend.

Mental health awareness programmes have been developed largely in countries other than the UK, such as Australia (e.g. Patton *et al.*, 2000). Some of these programmes have focused on specific problems, especially alcohol abuse (Komro *et al.*, 2001) and depression (Clarke *et al.*, 1993). A broad school-based mental health programme in Pakistan resulted in considerably improved mental health in school children who received the intervention (Rahman *et al.*, 1998). Some studies have produced less positive results (e.g. Clarke *et al.*, 1993), but the size of such studies has usually been so small that they were likely to have been underpowered to find an effect.

Approaches to school-based mental health promotion include a range of different types of intervention. Some are class-based and aimed at delivering a specific curriculum to all children in the class, others aim to change the ethos of the school, i.e. a whole-school approach, and others combine both class and whole-school approaches. The content of school-based mental health promotion interventions also varies greatly. Some programmes aim to teach pupils techniques that can help them to understand that there are many different ways of thinking about or reacting to problems, perhaps by focusing on specific behaviours, skills or environmental or cultural factors. A systematic review of the effects of mental health promotion programmes in schools was carried out by Wells and colleagues (2003). The results of this review suggest that the most successful interventions were those that were provided continuously over extensive periods of time, i.e. a year or more. Although the evidence was limited, they also found support for whole-school approaches that aim to involve everyone associated with the school, including pupils, staff, families and the community, as well as trying to change the environment and culture of the school.

There is a need for development and evaluation of school-based mental health awareness programmes in the UK. In our schools study, many respondents reported that although they could, and had, turned to friends when faced with problems, relatively few reported feeling comfortable about talking to their teachers about things that really bothered them. Furthermore, other researchers (e.g. Esters *et al.*, 1998) have noted that although the school counsellor is in the front line for providing assistance, very few students indicate that they have used this resource or other trained professionals for help with emotional problems. Instead, most have just turned to friends and family. Indeed, it is well known that mental health service resources designed to assist those in need of care are underutilised. One factor thought to contribute to this is the stigma attached to mental illness and the associated help-seeking process. Esters and colleagues (1998) suggested that the logical step in removing the stigma and thus removing an obstacle to service delivery would be to promote positive attitudes about seeking psychological help and to point out that adolescence is a prime time to attempt this. We suggest therefore that as part of a whole-school mental health awareness programme, there should be a focus on the key factors that are known to be important with regard to development and prevention of mental health problems in adolescents. The following therefore seem to be appropriate components:

PROBLEM-SOLVING SKILLS

The importance of developing effective problem-solving skills should be focused on, and adolescents should be given the opportunity to identify and try out different problem-solving strategies in the safe environment of the classroom. This might be in response to case vignettes.

SELF-ESTEEM

A simple explanation of what self-esteem is and why it is important should be provided. Pupils should then be taught how to measure their self-esteem along with simple strategies for countering negative thoughts and improving how they feel about themselves.

COPING WITH STRESS

Although adolescence is not necessarily a period of intense turmoil, it is a time of potential stress related to rapid and dramatic physical, hormonal, cognitive and psychological changes. It is important therefore for adolescents to recognise the symptoms of stress and to learn how to implement different strategies for coping with it.

AWARENESS OF MENTAL HEALTH PROBLEMS

Awareness of what mental health problems are and how to recognise whether someone (self or others) is experiencing such problems are important skills for adolescents to learn. This clearly needs to be at a simple level, but it should include how to recognise whether oneself or someone else is depressed or anxious. This seems particularly pertinent since, as we have emphasised, adolescents are more likely to turn to peers than to adults for help with their problems.

SEEKING HELP AND HELPING OTHERS

Different strategies for seeking help when adolescents are faced with emotional problems (either their own or a peer's) should be outlined. It is particularly important to explore with adolescents about when and how to break a confidence in order to get help from an adult for a friend who is at risk. It is also vital to highlight the different sources of support that are available to adolescents, with guidance on which source is best for which type of problem.

Secondary prevention

The goal of secondary prevention is to prevent an already existing condition from progressing. Therefore, the goal in relation to self-harming behaviour would be to identify those adolescents who are either experiencing thoughts of self-harm or suicidal ideation or who are at risk of or already engaging in deliberate self-harm, with a view to referring these adolescents for treatment. Proactive approaches, such as screening programmes, that focus on identifying adolescents most at risk for suicidal behaviour have been suggested by a number of authors (e.g. Garfinkel, 1989; Reynolds, 1991; Reynolds and Mazza, 1994; Shaffer et al., 1988).

Screening programmes

A variety of approaches using direct assessment have been proposed for identifying adolescents at risk (Miller and DuPaul, 1996). One approach involves a comprehensive class or school-wide screening focusing on pupils' global behaviours and overall well-being. This may include responses to questionnaires by pupils, their teachers, their parents and their peers. This is costly in terms of the time and effort required from many individuals. An alternative method is to focus on a narrower range of behaviours associated more closely with suicidal behaviour. This would also initially involve the screening of a class or whole school, followed up by individual interviews with those considered to be at risk.

A well-known screening programme that specifically targets at-risk individuals in schools is the Columbia Teen Screen (Shaffer et al., 1996). This programme elicits information on mood disorders, substance abuse and suicidal ideation and behaviour. It involves three stages of screening. In the first stage, all students complete a brief self-report questionnaire in class. Those identified as having abnormal scores then complete the Diagnostic Interview Schedule for Children (Shaffer and Gould, 2000). The third stage involves a face-to-face interview with a clinician, which will determine the need for referral for treatment or further evaluation. This programme has been running since 1996, has been found to be efficient and is now operating in over 45 sites in the USA (Shaffer and Craft, 1999).

Similarly, Reynolds (1991) has proposed a two-stage process of identifying young people who are actively thinking about killing themselves that uses both his Suicidal Ideation Questionnaire (Reynolds, 1987) and his Suicidal Behaviors Interview (Reynolds, 1990). The first stage involves all the young people in a school completing the Suicidal Ideation Questionnaire, which is designed to evaluate whether or not they are experiencing thoughts about suicide. A significant proportion of adolescents are likely to be identified; for example, in our schools study, 15 per cent of our sample indicated that they had had thoughts of self-harm in the previous year (in addition to 6.9% who reported actual self-harm). These adolescents are then invited to have a clinical interview to allow further evaluation of their suicidal status. Reynolds acknowledges that conducting clinical interviews on a large number of young people can be costly in terms of time and resources but suggests that this cost is small 'given the potential outcomes of not evaluating the suicidal status of young people who are thinking of killing themselves' (Reynolds, 1991: p.68).

Concerns about screening exist. For example, timing is important. Students at low risk of suicide at one screening may be at high risk a month later. Furthermore, because the signs indicating that an adolescent may engage in some form of suicidal behaviour can lack specificity (the signs are common in non-suicidal teens and include sadness, irritability and social withdrawal), there may be many false-positive cases. The referral of false-positives (pupils who are not truly at high risk of suicide or self-harm but who nonetheless score in the danger zone of the instrument) can be expensive and problematic and risks stigmatisation, both by the individuals themselves and by peers. Schools are also faced with the difficult decision of whether, when and how often to screen their pupils.

Beautrais and colleagues (1997) are clear in that they do *not* recommend the use of screening instruments in schools for the identification of young people at risk of suicide. Instead, they recommend that all teachers and, to a lesser extent, other school staff receive initial training to enable them to identify common signs that would prompt them to refer an individual to a counsellor. We would largely concur with this view, regarding screening as not very appropriate in the UK. However, the appropriateness of screening may depend partly on cultural values and attitudes.

Peer identification of at-risk adolescents

Even though adolescents see their peers as a key source of support, there is the important question of the extent to which they are able to recognise when friends are having difficulties and provide help, either themselves or through involving other people. This may seem a large burden to place on adolescents, but clearly if they are the main potential source of help for troubled peers then they need help in managing this important role. As a result, it is important to consider that vulnerable young people may be taking responsibility for some adolescents who are very disturbed and who might challenge the resources of even experienced mental health workers.

Intervention strategies that rely on peer helpers have been reviewed by Gould and colleagues (2003), who noted that the role that peers play varies considerably by programme, with some peers listening and reporting any possible warning signs and others taking on counselling responsibilities. Evaluations of these programmes are limited and often confined to student satisfaction measures. Potential negative side effects have not been explored. Indeed, Lewis and Lewis (1996) note that there is not yet a sufficient body of evidence documenting the efficacy or safety of peer-helping programmes, despite their widespread use, at least in the USA.

Tertiary prevention: dealing with the aftermath

All schools are likely at some stage to have at least one student seriously attempt suicide or die by suicide. When this happens, there will be consequences for other students. Many students will experience intense emotions of grief, guilt and anger as they try to understand and make sense of what may seem an inexplicable act. For some, it may bring back memories and reactions to other loss experiences. Perhaps most worryingly, for a small number of pupils, especially those who may already be experiencing difficulties, it may raise awareness of suicide as an option for them. Adolescents seem to be particularly vulnerable to the 'contagious' influence of suicide. For example, research has shown that in general there is a significant association between suicidal phenomena and exposure to suicide attempts in family members (Statham et al., 1998). As we have noted already, there are also very strong links between deliberate self-harm and exposure to acts of self-harm by friends. This can give rise to the clustering of suicides that has been known to occur in this age group (Gould et al. 1989, 1994). Indeed, Gould et al. (1994) suggest that the 'relative risk for suicide given exposure to the suicide of one or more other persons may be quite great'. These findings have clear implications for how the occurrence of suicidal behaviour in schools is managed. As a result, the guidelines put together by Beautrais and colleagues (1997) emphasise the importance of having a traumatic incident response plan. The aim of this is to prepare staff for the impact of suicidal behaviour and to ensure that procedures are documented so that staff can follow them clearly, even though they themselves are likely to be experiencing difficult emotions. This should result in there being a quick coordinated direct response in the event of an incident.

Professionals who are involved with adolescents in the school setting must be aware that a suicide or suicide attempt within the school may have an impact on other pupils and that appropriate support mechanisms should be put in place for those who may also be at risk. A timely response to a suicide is thought to be likely to reduce subsequent morbidity and mortality in fellow students (Gould *et al.*, 2003). The major goals of such a programme are to assist the survivors in the grief process, identify and refer those who may be at risk following the suicide, and provide accurate information about suicide, while attempting to minimise suicide contagion and to implement a structure for ongoing prevention efforts (Gould *et al.*, 2003; Underwood and Dunne-Maxim, 1997).

Hazell (1991) implemented postvention strategies in three schools in Australia after pupils had committed suicide. The strategies employed in the three schools were very similar, with adolescents who were considered most at risk and those who were closest to the deceased being asked to take part in a group discussion reflecting on the deceased and what they knew and how they had responded to the event. The difficulty of predicting suicide was explained with the aim of alleviating guilt. Symptoms of mental health problems were described, and the importance of seeking help from a responsible adult was emphasised, with certain members of the school staff agreeing to take responsibility for monitoring those considered to be most at risk. Although the impact of the programmes was not investigated in a systematic way, staff from the three schools reported that pupils were more prepared to present their difficulties to school staff in that there had been an increase in pupils presenting with distress and suicidal ideation in the subsequent months. They also seemed more willing to identify other pupils who appeared to be at risk.

The problem with postvention programmes is that evaluation is sparse. However, Gould and colleagues (2003) identified what they describe as a 'small and methodologically limited, yet encouraging study' by Poijula and colleagues (2001). They found that no new suicides took place during a four-year follow-up period in schools where adequate intervention took place, whereas the number of suicides increased significantly in schools after suicides with no adequate subsequent crisis intervention.

It is equally important for professionals who are involved with adolescents in the school setting to be aware that deliberate self-harm is a relatively common occurrence: 6.9 per cent of the adolescents who took part in our schools study reported having carried out an act of deliberate self-harm that met our study criteria in the previous year. In England, the Oxfordshire Adolescent Self-Harm Forum (2004), has produced guidelines that are written with the aim of helping school staff to support young people who harm themselves; an adapted version of these guidelines can be found in Appendix III. The guidelines begin by outlining what self-harm is and what might trigger episodes of self-harm. A number of alternative coping strategies for young people are suggested, including writing, drawing and talking about feelings, listening to loud music, drawing red lines on the skin with a washable pen, and putting an elastic band around the wrist, which can be snapped to cause pain. The main part of the guidelines focuses on how a member of school staff can help. Ethical issues such as confidentiality are discussed, and practical suggestions are put forward, such as how to manage a meeting with the young person who self-harms, the provision of a sample letter that can be sent to the parents/guardians of the young person and a sample incident form that can be completed when a young person self-harms on the school premises.

Summary and implications

In this chapter, we have focused on school-based initiatives for the prevention of suicidal behaviour. We have argued that schools are well placed to provide intervention and prevention programmes. We have suggested that rather than focusing on suicidal behaviour alone, a more appropriate approach would be to raise awareness about mental health issues in general. Thus, a successful mental health programme will include a focus on addressing and managing the difficulties faced by young people and equipping them with the skills to cope. This must include attention to recognising problems in peers and the best ways of helping them. Furthermore, such a programme should also involve the school staff to ensure that they have an awareness of the nature of psychiatric disorders and the pressures and problems that young people face, as well as the potential resources and sources of help, both for the adolescents and themselves. In the next chapter, we explore the role that the health service can play in the management and prevention of deliberate self-harm and suicidal behaviour among adolescents.

CHAPTER 7

The Health Service and Deliberate Self-harm

Introduction

As we discussed in Chapter 5, there is clear evidence from a number of sources to indicate that a substantial proportion of adolescents who carry out acts of deliberate self-harm or have thoughts of self-harm do not receive help. One important aspect of this issue is the attitude of young people to help-seeking, especially those adolescents who have problems. For example, in a study of adolescents in New Zealand, fewer of those who had thoughts of self-harm said they would seek professional help than did their peers who were not experiencing such problems but who were asked what they would do if they did have thoughts of self-harm (Carlton and Deane, 2000). In our schools study, a quarter of the adolescents who self-harmed did not think that they had a serious problem. This confirms Saunders and colleagues' (1994) finding that suggests that adolescents may need help in order to identify their problems and assess their severity. Furthermore, compared with their peers, adolescents in our study who reported deliberate self-harm or thoughts of self-harm indicated fewer categories of people with whom they felt able to talk about things that really bothered them. For most of those with a deliberate self-harm episode, at least one person or source knew about it, but over 20 per cent said that no one knew.

Another important aspect of the provision of help for adolescents with emotional problems and who may be at risk of deliberate self-harm concerns the availability of services. The document *Bridging the Gaps: Healthcare for Adolescents* (Royal College of Paediatrics and Child Health, 2003) provides an overview of the healthcare of adolescents in the UK and describes some of the current deficiencies. For example, there is a relative dearth of specific or discrete services for young people. It is of paramount importance that healthcare providers engage with young people with a view to (i) developing services that meet their needs and (ii) recognising that adolescent medicine is not so much about a particular set of diseases, but rather is concerned with the ways in which services are provided. In particular, the document highlights concerns that have been raised by adolescents that relate to access, confidentiality and privacy as well as the expertise and continuity of professionals and the settings in which care is provided. Of these issues, maintaining confidentiality is the prime concern that young people have reported as affecting their use of health services (Finlay, 1998). This concern about confidentiality, together with a lack of immediate access to family doctor services, may lead young people to use a range of other care providers, including walk-in medical centres, school health nurses, family planning services, and so on, which can mean that there is a lack of continuity in care. Alternatively, young people may not use formal sources of help at all.

Another problem regarding care for older adolescents (ages 16–18 years) is that this is the age at which there is a transition in services, from those for children and adolescents to those for adults. Differences in criteria between services for age limits for acceptance of referrals, combined with the general problems that may occur in transfer of care between services as adolescents reach the lower threshold for the adult service, can add further barriers to their receiving uninterrupted care.

Seeking help and using support systems are thought to have a buffering effect on reactions to stress, which can result in better adjustment and fewer emotional and behavioural problems (Raviv et al., 2000; Schonert-Reichl and Muller, 1996). However, as we have already pointed out, many adolescents are poor at utilising these formal sources of help and, instead, prefer to turn to their informal networks of friends (especially) and family for support, help and guidance. In this chapter, we consider the role that the health service and other agencies can play in managing and preventing deliberate self-harm in adolescents. We discuss the implications of the findings from our schools study and focus in particular on the role of general practitioner services, hospital emergency departments and psychiatric services.

General practitioner services

In the UK, on average a general practitioner (GP) will experience suicide in one of his or her patients only every four to five years. Deliberate self-harm resulting in hospital presentation will occur in approximately four to eight patients per year, but this number may be greater for GPs serving areas characterised by socioeconomic deprivation and social fragmentation (Hawton *et al.*, 2001). About a quarter of such patients will be teenagers. However, as our schools study has shown, deliberate self-harm is far more common in adolescents than is represented by hospital presentation statistics, with 6.9 per cent reporting deliberate self-harm in the previous year and only one in eight going to hospital as a result. Most of those who did not go to hospital did not reach the attention of any health professionals. It may, therefore, be difficult for many health professionals to recognise deliberate self-harm in young people as a significant problem. This section of the chapter focuses on how GPs can identify that an adolescent patient is at risk of deliberate self-harm, what GPs should do and how GP services for adolescents can be improved.

Recognising the problem and the role of the general practitioner

It is known that up to two-thirds of all suicide attempters identified in hospital samples have visited their GP shortly before the act (Hawton and Blackstock, 1976; Michel *et al.*, 1997; Van Casteren *et al.*, 1993), although this proportion may be lower in teenagers. Furthermore, there is an increase in the frequency of visits to GPs before engaging in suicidal behaviour (Appleby *et al.*, 1996; Michel *et al.*, 1997). This suggests that the reasons for the individual visiting the GP are likely to be related to the development of a suicidal crisis.

However, even when an individual contacts his or her GP, the individual does not always communicate his or her thoughts of deliberate self-harm and tends to focus instead on physical health symptoms. For example, a study of suicide in young people conducted by Hawton and colleagues (1999a) found that 78.4 per cent of subjects aged under 25 years had seen their GP within the last year of their life. Of these, 35 per cent had seen their GP in the month before their death. In terms of expressing suicidal thoughts, 44.3 per cent had expressed such thoughts within the month before death. Most commonly, these were expressed to relatives (24.7%) followed by professionals, including GPs (20.1%). Thus there are two problems. First, people may simply not visit their GPs; second, if an individual does visit his or her GP, it may be that the individual finds it difficult to talk to his or her doctor about emotional problems because of feeling ashamed or fearing being stigmatised and so prefering to focus on physical health problems (Michel, 2000). There is also the difficulty that even if the problem is identified, then the GP may not know how best to manage it or there may be limited or inadequate secondary care services.

Michel (2000) suggests that GPs should be trained using a model that considers suicide attempts and other self-harming behaviour that come to medical attention as the tip of an iceberg. This is in keeping with the findings concerning hospital presentation of deliberate self-harm in our schools study (see Chapter 3 and Figure 3.4). The major part of the iceberg, which may be largely invisible to the GP, represents deliberate self-harm that does not come to medical attention plus suicidal thoughts and emotional crises. The importance of the model is that it highlights graphically the need for prevention of deliberate self-harm and suicide to start by recognising the (often covert) signs of emotional problems.

Adolescents as a group require special consideration as users of health services. This is something that has been recognised for a considerable amount of time. Adolescents may lack confidence in simply accessing primary healthcare services; once they do access services, they may lack the ability to communicate how they are feeling. As a result, it has been suggested that GPs should try to establish whether there are underlying psychosocial reasons for an individual's physical symptoms. One way of doing this is to ask simple open questions, such as 'How are you getting on with life?' This signifies to the individual that the GP is there to listen to them and that psychosocial aspects of health problems will be considered in the consultation. It is important that the GP follows up the adolescent's response to make clear that all aspects of the adolescent's life are included in the question. If an adolescent identifies problem area(s), then the GP could refer to the list we used in our schools study to focus on specific areas of concern identified by the adolescent. Furthermore, if the GP suspects that an adolescent is engaging in deliberate self-harm or is thinking about self-harm, then we recommend that the GP asks the adolescent directly about these behaviours. Useful questions are:

- Have you seriously thought about taking an overdose or trying to harm yourself but not actually done so?

- Have you worked out any specific plans for trying to harm yourself?

- Have you ever deliberately taken an overdose or tried to harm yourself in some way?

- When was the last time you took an overdose or tried to harm yourself?

- Describe what you did on that occasion.

- Describe in your own words why you think you took an overdose or tried to harm yourself on that occasion.

Improving general practitioner services for adolescents

Recognising the problem of adult suicidal behaviour is difficult for GPs, because many patients prefer to focus on physical rather than emotional health issues. Adolescents bring their own problems and, unfortunately, some GPs do not recognise the health concerns and needs of young people. In addition, recognition of mental health problems and their contribution to physical symptoms may be limited (Kramer and Garralda, 1998). Therefore, this section focuses on how GP services could be improved to address the specific issues that concern adolescents.

As noted above, a key issue that young people have reported as influencing their use of health services concerns confidentiality (Finlay, 1998). The Royal College of Paediatrics and Child Health (2003: p.45) has suggested that this issue can be 'minimised by making general practitioner practices "friendly" for young people, addressing issues of family doctor confidentiality, copying in young people on clinical correspondence and, perhaps, the holding of personal health records by young people'. Other suggestions have been highlighted in the leaflet *Getting it Right for Teenagers in Your Practice* (Royal College of General Practitioners and Royal College of Nursing, 2002), which is available from the Royal College of General Practitioners. The leaflet was circulated to all general practices in England, with the intention of raising awareness of issues of teenage health and access to primary care. It contains a scoring system to self-assess 'teenage-friendliness'. The scoring criteria focus on a number of issues, including whether the practice has a written confidentiality policy for young people, whether the practice displays magazines and information leaflets aimed at young people, whether the practice GPs see young people under the age of 16 years without a parent being present, whether practice staff are trained to be teenage-friendly, and whether the practice runs clinics especially for young people. It is planned that these criteria for young people's services will become part of the quality points system within primary care in England as well as being rolled out by commissioners of young people's services to help deliver the National Service Framework for Children and Young People (Department of Health, 2004).

Fostering young people's independence and sense of responsibility for their health is also important. Until young people reach adolescence, they tend to present to health services with a parent and have not had to access the services by themselves. Adolescents could, therefore, be considered as 'new' users of healthcare services and, as such, their developing autonomy needs to be encouraged by professionals, perhaps enabling them to spend part of a consultation without their parents present. It is important to note that young people are likely to be learning about how to access and use services appropriately and so may have different perceptions compared with their parents or professionals regarding healthcare. As a result, a young person's initial contact with a service may be the last if it is not perceived by him or her to have been appropriate. Thus, two key strategies are essential: GP services should begin to inform young people about the services that they can access before they need them, and GPs should start to see young people on their own as a routine for part of the consultation when they come in with a parent, as a means of building a relationship that the young person trusts.

Under certain circumstances, a primary care team member might feel that an adolescent is sufficiently at risk that his or her parents or guardians should be informed. It is helpful if the GP clarifies this when seeing young people with emotional problems. If the GP is considering overriding confidentiality and disclosing information to a parent or another professional, then they should discuss this with the adolescent first in a sensitive and respectful manner, acknowledging that this may be difficult for the young person but emphasising that there is a need to keep him or her safe. The threshold for discussing information with parents will need to be lower with younger adolescents. It is important to bear in mind that in the UK, under the Children Act 1989 (HMSO, 1989), parents have a responsibility to be 'parental' towards their children. Therefore, they may need to be given information in order to provide appropriate parenting. This has to be weighed up against the young person's right to confidentiality.

Assessing adolescent mental health problems

The major burden of assessing and managing adolescent mental health problems falls to primary care practitioners. Health-risk behaviours cluster together, and the young person's health is associated strongly with many important health outcomes (Viner and MacFarlane, 2005). Indeed, the recognition, evaluation and treatment of mental health problems and related suicidal or self-harming behaviour is described as the highest priority in adolescent health (Michaud and Fombonne, 2005). However, identifying, treating and following up such mental health and emotional problems in young people can be complicated for a number of reasons, not least because problems may be dismissed as simply reflecting adolescent turmoil. It is, therefore, important that GPs are made aware of the emotional and mental health problems that have been shown to be linked significantly with deliberate self-harm.

In Chapter 4, we presented evidence to show that depression, anxiety, self-esteem and impulsivity were linked significantly to self-harm in adolescents. We suggest that the scales we used in our schools study could be useful tools to assist in the assessment of adolescents' levels of depression, anxiety, self-esteem, stressful life events and self-reported deliberate self-harm and suicidal ideation.

In terms of measuring adolescents' levels of depression and anxiety, we suggest using the Hospital Anxiety and Depression Scale (Zigmond and Snaith, 1983). This has been validated for use with adolescents by White and colleagues (1999). It is a short, 14-question, user-friendly, reliable scale designed to assess levels of depression and anxiety in non-psychiatric populations. Adolescents are asked to think about how they have been feeling recently and in response to each question to tick a box that best describes how they have been feeling in the past week. Two examples of questions from the scale are: 'I feel tense and wound up', with response options of 'Most of the time', 'A lot of the time', 'Time to time – occasionally' and 'Not at all', and 'I have lost interest in my appearance', with response of 'Definitely', 'I don't take so much care as I should', 'I may not take quite as much care' and 'I take just as much care as ever'. When scoring the responses, GPs could use cut-off points (White *et al.*, 1999) to identify adolescents for whom depression and/or anxiety may be a particular concern. It is also essential to assess specific signs and symptoms that should be looked for in order to investigate whether adolescents are suffering from anxiety, depression or other psychiatric disorders.

In our schools study, we also used a shortened eight-item version of Robson's Self-concept Scale (Robson, 1989) to measure the adolescents' levels of self-esteem (Appendix IV). In this scale, adolescents are asked to think about how they feel most of the time and, in light of this, to indicate how much they agree or disagree with each of the eight statements. Response options include 'Completely disagree', 'Disagree', 'Agree' and 'Completely agree'. Three examples of questions are: 'I am glad I am who I am', 'There are lots of things I would change about myself if I could' and 'Everyone seems much more confident and contented than me'. While there are no cut-off points for scores on this version of the scale, the general pattern of responses will provide a good impression of how a young person feels about him- or herself.

It is unclear how best we should assess impulsivity. We used a shortened version of the Plutchik Impulsivity Scale (Plutchik and Van Praag, 1986). For the GP, it may be best to ask adolescents how far they agree with a few simple statements such as: 'I plan ahead', 'I do things on the spur of the moment' and 'I find it difficult to control my emotions'.

We have already suggested how GPs might ask adolescents about thoughts of self-harm. Adolescents thought to be at risk should also be asked about their experience of suicidal behaviour among their family and friends. Furthermore, the GP should ask adolescents carefully about their alcohol and drug use. In addition, the GP should enquire about family relationships and the level of support currently available from family members. If the adolescent has already carried out an act of deliberate self-harm, then the GP should, in addition to assessing the physical severity of the act, enquire about the possible reasons and motives for self-harm. These aspects of self-harm were discussed in detail in Chapter 3. Other aspects of the assessment are considered later in this chapter.

What general practitioners can do when they detect adolescents at risk

Having discussed the difficulties of identifying and assessing adolescent mental health problems that face primary care practitioners, we now turn to considering what GPs can do if they detect adolescents at risk. Evidence as to how a GP can best manage patients who have deliberately harmed themselves is currently lacking. Bennewith and colleagues (2002) explored the effectiveness of a GP intervention designed to prevent repeat episodes of deliberate self-harm. The intervention used guidelines developed by consulting a group consisting of GPs with an interest in mental health, psychiatrists, a psychologist, a specialist nurse, a voluntary worker from Samaritans and patients with a history of deliberate self-harm. The research team synthesised the views of the group to produce the final version of the guidelines (Sharp *et al.*, 2003). Although the intervention was not found to make a difference to the incidence of repeat episodes of deliberate self-harm, the guidelines can be thought of as a useful educational tool for GPs, who often lack formal training in the management of deliberate self-harm.

Although the guidelines were not aimed specifically at adolescents, the key points are applicable to them. In terms of the general management of people who engage in deliberate self-harm the first step is to ask the patient what he or she thinks is needed. In addition, GPs should consider regular monitoring of the patient's mental health and should discuss strategies that the individual can implement as a means of coping with the urge to engage in deliberate self-harm, such as talking to a trusted person, engaging in distracting or relaxing activities, taking exercise, listening to music or going out with peers. It is also reasonable to expect GPs to be able to teach simple problem-solving strategies. Family members may also be encouraged to ensure that there are supportive family relationships.

The GP should stress the 24-hour availability of GP services and also the availability of other crisis services, e.g. telephone helplines. In addition, GPs should treat any associated disorders that have been identified, including anxiety and depression and problems with alcohol and drugs.

The first line of treatment by the GP should involve provision of support for the adolescent, either by the GP or by a suitable member of the practice team. Simple psychological therapy such as problem-solving and/or family meetings should be considered. The GP can also direct the adolescent towards appropriate self-help resources.

If the problems are severe, and/or the adolescent may be at risk, and/or initial attempts at helping have been unsuccessful and the GP feels that management of the problems is beyond his or her capabilities or knowledge, then the GP should refer the adolescent on to other services. In the UK, these include primary care child and adolescent mental health teams. For the most severe problems, referral to a secondary-level child and adolescent mental health team will be more appropriate. Finally, the GP should discuss the need for further follow-up with the patient, whether with the GP again, a primary care nurse, a mental health professional, a voluntary organisation or social services.

General hospital emergency services

Increasing numbers of adolescents access general hospital emergency departments, rather than primary healthcare facilities, especially for sexual health, mental health, self-harm and substance use issues. However, few if any emergency departments in England currently have specific provision for young people. This is not necessarily in itself a problem. What is important, however, is to ensure that all staff possess the skills to communicate and deal effectively with challenging young people. The Royal College of Paediatrics and Child Health (2003) suggests that all those who work in emergency departments should have some basic training in adolescent health.

The emergency department provides the main medical service for people who have engaged in deliberate self-harm. This is a very common reason for hospital presentation. In the 1990s, it was estimated that 170,000 cases of deliberate self-harm by people of all ages presented to hospital each year in the UK (Kapur *et al.*, 1998). Due to increases in rates of self-harm, the figure at the time of writing is probably considerably higher. Between 20,000 and 30,000 of these individuals will be adolescents. The majority of episodes involve self-poisoning, but the other frequent method of deliberate self-harm is self-cutting. The extent to which people who engage in deliberate self-harm wish to die can vary greatly, and level of suicidal intent is often not reflected in the physical danger of the act (Beck *et al.*, 1975; Browne *et al.*, 2004). Careful assessment of each individual is of paramount importance (National Institute for Clinical Excellence, 2004; Royal College of Psychiatrists, 1998).

Although, as we demonstrated clearly in our schools study, many acts of deliberate self-harm by adolescents do not come to the attention of clinicians, the number of adolescents, especially girls, attending emergency departments with deliberate self-harm has increased over the past couple of decades (Hawton *et al.*, 2003b). The treatment an individual receives on arrival at the general hospital varies widely, in spite of well-established standards published by the Royal College of Psychiatrists (2004). Nearly half of all hospital attendances in England by adults following self-harm do not lead to a specialist assessment (Gunnell *et al.*, 2005). Furthermore, whether a patient receives a psychological assessment varies greatly between hospitals;

the percentages in a recent study of a representative sample of hospitals ranged from as low as 36 per cent to an upper figure of 82 per cent (Bennewith *et al.*, 2004). Patients who are managed entirely in the emergency department without admission to a general hospital bed are especially unlikely to receive a psychosocial assessment. For example, in a report focusing on deliberate self-harm in Oxford, it was noted that more than two-thirds of non-admitted patients were not assessed (Hawton *et al.*, 2003b) and, therefore, were not usually offered any further help.

The guideline published by the National Institute for Clinical Excellence (2004) proposes that all deliberate self-harm patients under the age of 16 years should be admitted overnight to allow full psychosocial assessment the following day. The National Institute for Clinical Excellence (NICE) guideline also encourages the use of the Australian Mental Health Triage Scale for when deliberate self-harm patients arrive at a general hospital. This is a comprehensive scale that provides an effective means of rating clinical urgency so that patients are seen in a timely manner. The scale has five levels:

- Category 1 is classified as 'emergency', where the person's condition is immediately life-threatening; for example, the patient may have taken an overdose and be unresponsive.

- Category 2 is also classified as 'emergency': the patient is violent, aggressive, suicidal and a danger to self and/or others and has/may have a police escort.

- Category 3 is classified as 'urgent': the patient is very distressed or psychotic, is likely to become aggressive, is a danger to self and/or others, and is experiencing a situational crisis.

- Category 4 is classified as 'semi-urgent': the patient has a long-standing semi-urgent mental disorder/problem.

- Category 5 is classified as 'non-urgent': the patient has a long-standing non-acute mental disorder/problem.

The scale was developed by Smart and colleagues (1999) to address the fact that triage was traditionally related to physical injury and illness and was not easily adaptable to mental health presentations. This meant that people experiencing mental health problems tended to receive low triage priority, which in turn meant that they faced longer waiting times, which was thought to contribute to a high incidence of these people leaving the emergency department without being seen (Happell *et al.*, 2003; Heslop *et al.*,

2000; Smart *et al.*, 1999). However, the majority of adolescents with deliberate self-harm will be classified in category 5 on the scale, or even lie outside the scale, because of their appearing largely to have interpersonal problems (although on detailed assessment (see p.144), symptoms of psychiatric disorder may be identified). Thus, it is somewhat questionable how useful this scale is for prioritising adolescents who present with deliberate self-harm.

In addition to the immediate assessment of the medical consequences of self-poisoning or self-injury, a brief assessment of the patient's psychiatric status and risk should be conducted. This should not be delayed until after medical treatment has been completed, unless life-saving medical treatment is needed or the patient is otherwise incapable of being assessed. In particular, it is important to determine whether the person has a serious psychiatric disorder such as severe depression or psychosis and whether the person is actively suicidal. Potential methods of self-harm such as tablets and sharp objects should be removed, and staff should be aware that the patient may try to leave before a psychiatric assessment has been conducted (Fox and Hawton, 2004).

There is clearly a need for emergency department staff to have basic skills in assessment and for them to be able to readily obtain urgent psychiatric assessment when they judge it to be necessary. In particular, clinicians should take full account of the distress and emotional disturbance experienced by people who self-harm, in addition to the physical effects of the overdose or injury itself.

It is of paramount importance that a full psychiatric assessment takes place only when the patient has recovered from any toxic effects of his or her act of deliberate self-harm. The consequences of not adhering to this guidance are that assessing an individual's mental state can be compromised and he or she may show distorted or impaired recall of events. Of course, an earlier assessment of mental state will be required if the patient appears to be disturbed or severely distressed.

At one time, the psychosocial assessment of people who engaged in deliberate self-harm was regarded as the responsibility primarily of psychiatrists. However, increases in the clinical responsibilities of non-medical clinical staff and the findings of research have resulted in a major change in the pattern of services in the UK. Whatever the discipline of the staff members involved in this kind of role, it is of the utmost importance that they have background experience and skills in the management of people with emotional and psychiatric disorders as well as training in the assessment and treatment of people who engage in deliberate self-harm. We will now consider how psychosocial assessment of adolescents who have self-harmed might be conducted.

Assessment of adolescents who have deliberately self-harmed

As Hawton and Catalan (1987) have described, an optimum psychosocial assessment following an episode of deliberate self-harm should focus on a number of key areas. We have adapted this approach for use with adolescents. The topics to cover when assessing adolescents who have engaged in deliberate self-harm are as follows:

- Life events and problems preceding the event
- Suicidal intent
- Other motives for the act
- Psychiatric and personality characteristics
- Family history
- Alcohol and drug misuse
- Coping resources and supports
- Exposure to suicide and deliberate self-harm by others
- Risk of repetition and of suicide

The assessment should include at least one interview with the young person alone. In the interview, it is crucial to use whatever skills are necessary to engage the adolescent. It is also important to try to help the adolescent think differently about his or her problems and the possible solutions.

Adolescents over the age of 12 years can usually be interviewed in much the same way as adults (Harrington, 2001). Parents or other guardians, friends, teachers and other professionals involved in the care of the adolescent, including the GP, should be asked to provide information that can supplement that given by the adolescent.

Life events and problems preceding the event

Information concerning the adolescent's problems and the events that preceded the act of self-harm should be obtained during the interview. One way of doing this is to obtain a very detailed account of the few days leading up to the act. This will usually reveal major problems that the adolescent is facing. It is useful, however, to review briefly other potential problem areas. The following is a checklist of problem areas and other influences that may be associated with adolescent deliberate self-harm:

- family problems
- relationship problems
- school problems
- alcohol use
- drug use
- bullying
- physical abuse
- sexual abuse
- sexual orientation worries
- in trouble with the police
- having friends who have engaged in deliberate self-harm
- having a family member who has engaged in deliberate self-harm
- trauma, such as bereavement
- media and Internet influences.

Suicidal intent and other motives

Motives involved in deliberate self-harm should be assessed during the interview. The adolescent who has engaged in deliberate self-harm can be asked to explain why in his or her own words. In addition, a useful list of motives (see Chapter 2) has been developed based on research conducted on adults in the 1970s (Bancroft et al., 1976, 1979) and subsequently used by other researchers (e.g. Hawton et al., 1982a; Hjelmeland et al., 2002), including in adolescents (Rodham et al., 2004). This can be shown to the adolescent, who can then be asked to indicate which of the motives applied in his or her case and whether there were other motives not listed. It is best to do this after the adolescent has been asked to explain the intentions behind the act in his or her own words.

The clinician should also make his or her own assessment of the adolescent's likely motives. This is clearly a judgemental process. Clinicians often differ from adolescent self-harmers in their attribution of motives, with adolescents more often saying that they wanted to die and clinicians more often attributing motives concerning interpersonal communication such as to find out whether someone loved them or to try to change the behaviour of others (Hawton et al., 1982a). This does not mean that patients or clinicians are either right or wrong; it simply reflects differing appraisals of the act. For the clinician, the important thing is to feel that he or she has a motivational understanding for the act. If not, then the clinician should suspect that he or she is lacking certain information and/or that the patient has an undetected psychiatric disorder that was a major contributor to the act (Hawton and Catalan, 1987).

The level of suicidal intent, i.e. apparent wish to die, at the time of self-harm is an indicator of risk for later suicide (Harriss et al., 2005). It will also be of relevance to clinical decisions about aftercare and should, therefore, be measured routinely in clinical practice. Probably the best established instrument for assessing suicidal intent is the Beck Suicide Intent Scale (Beck et al., 1974), which consists of 15 questions in two sections. The first section (eight questions) concerns the circumstances of the act, e.g. whether the act was carried out in isolation, precautions taken to avoid discovery and whether the person had made preparations in the anticipation of his or her death. The second section (seven questions) includes items about the person's attitudes and feelings about the act, e.g. the anticipated outcome. Research has shown that high suicidal intent scores are associated with increased risk of suicide, especially in the first year after deliberate self-harm (Harriss et al., 2005). The circumstances section of the scale performs better in this respect than the self-report section. It is possible that items in the self-report section are more vulnerable to distortion by the patient, who might want to enhance the social desirability of the act or exaggerate the wish to die. However, as with other risk factors, the ability of the scale to predict risk in any individual patient is relatively low (Harriss and Hawton, 2005). In assessing risk, therefore, the clinician needs to take account of all the available information, including the specific circumstances of the individual patient.

Psychiatric and personality characteristics

Psychiatric disorders are common in adolescents who engage in deliberate self-harm (Burgess *et al.*, 1998; Kerfoot *et al.*, 1996) and add to their risk of repetition of self-harm (Hawton *et al.*, 1999b) and of suicide (Shaffer *et al.*, 1988). Such disorders are also a source of distress and are usually amenable to treatment. It is, therefore, essential that a careful assessment for symptoms or signs of psychiatric disorder be carried out. This is not easy, especially as variations in mood and behaviour are part of normal adolescence. Normal phenomena can be distinguished from more serious problems by their duration, persistence and impact of symptoms (Michaud and Fombonne, 2005). Assessments of these will require interviewing not only the adolescent but also parents and other informants, including school staff, and speaking to the adolescent's GP.

The main disorders likely to be found in adolescents who self-harm are depression, anxiety, substance misuse disorders, eating disorders, conduct disorder and attention deficit hyperactivity disorder (ADHD). Symptoms and behaviour that require further assessment include:

- signs of overt mood disturbance, e.g. low mood, tearfulness, loss of interest in usual activities
- physical complaints, e.g. headache, stomach ache, backache, sleep problems
- aggression and deviant behaviour, e.g. theft, damage to property
- isolation and loneliness
- deterioration in school performance or behaviour
- use of drugs and excessive consumption of alcohol
- weight loss or failure of normal weight gain with age.

During an assessment of possible depressive disorder, the adolescent should be asked about the symptoms listed in the World Health Organization (WHO) diagnostic criteria (World Health Organization, 1993), including:

- persistent sad or irritable mood
- loss of interest in activities

- loss of energy or tiring easily

- substantial change in aspect or body weight

- difficulty sleeping, including sleeping excessively

- psychomotor agitation or retardation

- feelings of worthlessness or inappropriate guilt

- difficulty concentrating

- recurrent thoughts of death or suicide.

Masked presentations of depression are common in adolescents, particularly in younger adolescents and boys. These include behavioural problems, substance misuse, school phobia or failure, fatigue and other physical symptoms (Michaud and Fombonne, 2005). In addition to asking about current and recent symptoms, the assessor should enquire about previous psychiatric or psychological problems and any treatment that has been received. The assessor should also ask whether there is a history of psychiatric disorder in the adolescent's parents or siblings.

Personality is very much in formation during adolescence. Clinicians are therefore reluctant to make diagnoses of personality disorder in adolescents, especially in younger individuals. It is, nevertheless, useful to enquire, especially through parents and other informants, about specific traits and psychological characteristics that may be relevant to deliberate self-harm. These include low self-esteem, impulsivity, hopelessness, aggression and difficulties with problem-solving (Kingsbury et al., 1999; Mann et al., 1999; Speckens and Hawton, 2005).

Family history

A family history of suicide has been shown to be associated with suicidal behaviour at all stages of the lifecycle. Adolescents are more likely to engage in suicidal behaviour when there is a lifetime family history of suicidal behaviour among first-degree relatives (Hawton et al., 2002; Pfeffer et al., 1998). It is, therefore, important for the clinician to establish whether there is a family history of suicidal behaviour. Specific questions include the following:

- Has anyone in your family attempted suicide or deliberately harmed themselves?

- Has anyone in your family died by suicide?

If the answer to either of these is positive, then the timing of the act or acts should be ascertained. It is also important to ask whether the adolescent believes that his or her family history, current family background and/or current family relationships and living arrangements had any effect on their decision to self-harm.

Alcohol and drug misuse

As we described in Chapter 4, several studies have identified associations between deliberate self-harm and alcohol and drug misuse. In our schools study, the risk of deliberate self-harm rose with increasing amounts of alcohol consumed. We also found drug use to be one of the stronger predictors of deliberate self-harm. Therefore, the adolescent's use of drugs and alcohol must be assessed. In terms of alcohol, adolescents might first be asked to report on the amount of alcohol that they normally consume during a 'typical week', followed by questions concerning the amount of alcohol consumed before the deliberate self-harm incident. They should also be asked about whether they have taken drugs, how often they do so and what kinds of drug they take. Responses to questions about alcohol and especially drug use may be guarded. More honest answers may result if the assessor conveys to the adolescent his or her recognition that alcohol and drug use is common in adolescence (but at the same time not making non-users feel 'abnormal'), indicates clearly the confidential nature of the interview and generally behaves in a non-judgemental manner.

Coping resources and supports

It is important to know what sources of help and support, including peer relationships, adolescents who engage in deliberate self-harm feel are available to them and what coping methods they use when they are feeling worried or upset about something. If adolescents are unable to communicate their problems and needs to others, then they are likely to be unable to obtain appropriate support. In our schools study, less than half (46.7%) of the adolescents who had engaged in deliberate self-harm reported that they had tried to get help beforehand.

It is important to find out with whom adolescents who engage in deliberate self-harm feel they can talk and to explore the barriers that prevent adolescents from seeking help. Such information provides the assessor with valuable information concerning the identification of potential sources of help that adolescents are not currently making use of. It also provides the assessor with an opportunity to address unhelpful or inaccurate assumptions that may prevent help-seeking.

In addition, exploring the kinds of coping strategies that adolescents who engage in deliberate self-harm employ can inform the planning of interventions that are more relevant to individual adolescents. We therefore recommend that in addition to exploring with whom the adolescent feels able to talk about things that worry or upset him or her, the assessor might also ask the adolescent to indicate what coping strategies the adolescent tends to use when faced with difficult situations. In Chapter 5, we discussed coping strategies that differentiated adolescents in our schools study who self-harmed from other adolescents. In summary, adolescents who self-harmed were more likely when faced with problems to engage in emotion-focused coping strategies, such as having an alcoholic drink or getting angry, and less likely to talk to someone or try to sort out their problems. Problem-focused coping is likely to be more effective than emotion-focused coping. Identifying the types of coping strategy an adolescent tends to use can, therefore, help the clinician to determine alternative styles of coping that the adolescent might be encouraged to use.

Assessing risk of repetition and suicide

As indicated earlier, repetition of deliberate self-harm is common (Owens *et al.*, 2002). Over half of the adolescents in our schools study with an episode of deliberate self-harm in the previous year had carried out more than one act. Repetition rates are lower in hospital samples, probably because of the high prevalence of self-poisoning. Self-cutting, which is more common in adolescents with self-harm who do not present to hospital, is repeated much more often. There is also a small but important subgroup of very frequent repeaters. The risk of suicide is high in those who repeatedly self-harm (Sakinofsky, 2000). Repetition of deliberate self-harm indicates persistent or recurrent psychosocial problems (Hawton *et al.*, 1999b). Repeaters of deliberate self-harm are also needy consumers of mental health and social services (Sakinofsky, 2000).

Estimation of the risk of repetition is therefore a very important part of the assessment. Various scales have been developed to predict repetition (e.g. Buglass and Horton, 1974; Kreitman and Foster, 1991). For adolescents, the key factors that have been identified as being associated with the risk of repetition of deliberate self-harm include previous episodes of self-harm, level of depression, psychosis, alcohol or drug misuse, history of sexual abuse, personality disorder, previous psychiatric treatment and chronic medical conditions (Hawton *et al.*, 1999b; Reith *et al.*, 2003; Vajda and Steinbeck, 2000). It is, however, important to remember that predictive factors are relatively crude, and so accurate prediction of risk of repetition is very difficult. Therefore, assessment must also include careful attention to each adolescent's unique characteristics and circumstances.

Increased risk of suicide following deliberate self-harm in young people is associated with male gender, older age, violent suicide attempts, bipolar and psychiatric disorders, substance misuse, previous psychiatric hospital admission and, especially, repetition of self-harm (Goldacre and Hawton, 1985; Hawton and Harriss, submitted; Otto, 1972). The same caveat about accuracy of prediction of repetition of self-harm applies even more strongly to prediction of risk of suicide, since the frequency of suicide is so much lower.

Another important factor to consider in the assessment of risk is possible access to dangerous methods that might be used in a suicidal act, such as an unlocked medical cabinet, sharp knives or guns (Brent *et al.*, 1987). Possible influences that may encourage suicidal behaviour, such as friends with a history of such acts and media and Internet influences, should also be enquired about.

Treatment options following deliberate self-harm

A key consideration in the management of the adolescent who has engaged in deliberate self-harm is whether psychiatric hospitalisation is required. Factors associated with the need for admission include severe psychiatric disorders, such as severe depression, bipolar disorder and schizophrenia, and high suicide risk.

For the majority of patients, treatment in the community will be indicated. Evidence is being gathered from studies of adults that shows that many patients may be helped by brief psychological treatment programmes (e.g. Guthrie *et al.*, 2001; Hawton *et al.*, 1997; Townsend *et al.*, 2001). In this section of this chapter, we focus on some of the forms of outpatient treatment that may be offered to adolescents who engage in deliberate self-harm.

Problem-solving therapy and crisis intervention

Studies of the psychological characteristics of adults who engage in deliberate self-harm have demonstrated that they have relatively poor problem-solving skills (e.g. Schotte and Clum, 1987), which therefore makes them more at risk of getting into crisis when faced by major stresses. In a recent review of the research literature on problem-solving skills in adolescents and their possible association with suicidal behaviour, evidence of deficits in problem-solving, especially in relation to social problems, was found for suicide attempters. However, where depression and/or hopelessness were controlled for, differences between such adolescents and control adolescents tended to be reduced (Speckens and Hawton, 2005). This suggests that depression may be a major factor that undermines problem-solving. More problem-solving deficits were found in adolescents with multiple episodes of self-harm than in those with single episodes. Williams and Pollock (2000) propose that, as a group, suicidal people may be less effective or more passive in solving problems in general. Clinicians should take account of any deficits in social problem-solving skills during the assessment and treatment of adolescents with suicidal behaviour.

Problem-solving therapy is based on the hypothesis that suicidal behaviour is due to an individual being deficient in psychological resources to resolve their problems. This may be due to depression and/or a long-standing paucity of effective coping strategies. Deficits in problem-solving shown by many individuals who harm themselves often appear to result from their having relatively few specific examples of problem-solving strategies, due to their tending to have overgeneralised autobiographical memory patterns (Williams and Pollock, 2000). These memory patterns are thought in many cases to have developed due to exposure to traumatic experiences during childhood or adolescence. Retention of non-specific memories may help to modify the emotions linked to these unpleasant experiences. However, this non-specific approach to stressful situations may generalise to other means of dealing with them. Where this is the case, one component of problem-solving therapy may be aimed at countering this tendency.

Another characteristic of the problem-solving ability of people who engage in self-harm is that they tend to adopt a passive approach to solving problems (Linehan et al., 1987). In problem-solving therapy, the therapist tries to counteract this style by requiring the patient to take a very active role in identifying and understanding problems and generating and implementing adaptive solutions.

Hawton and Kirk (1989) describe problem-solving therapy in some detail. This approach is central to crisis intervention. In short, the therapy can be divided into three phases: analysing the problem, generating and evaluating potential solutions, and implementing the solutions. In the first phase, the therapist will help the patient to articulate the problem and in so doing encourage the patient to define the problem and assess and understand the different factors that contribute to it.

During the second phase, the therapist helps the patient to generate solutions to the problem. Williams and Pollock (2000) highlight the fact that suicidal patients have difficulty in generating alternative solutions, which is thought to be related to the cognitive rigidity that characterises these patients. Therapists will need to encourage the patient to think of as many different options as possible, including those that may seem extreme. Once potential solutions are generated, the patient is then encouraged to evaluate them and to choose the most effective solutions.

Finally, the therapist will coach the patient in implementing the chosen solutions to the patient's problems. This is done by carrying out the solutions both cognitively and behaviourally and allows the identification of any potential obstacles to the implementation of the strategy. Cognitive therapy techniques are employed to help the patient understand blocks to carrying out the tasks, such as low motivation and pessimism about achieving success, and also identification of new strategies where earlier strategies have proved unsuccessful, including renegotiation of goals.

Cognitive behaviour therapy

A key principle of cognitive behaviour therapy is that the ways in which a person interprets events and experiences have major effects on the person's mood and behaviour. Some individuals develop automatic patterns of thinking that are considered to be distortions of reality. These patterns may result from states of depression and anxiety, and they are also likely to worsen such disorders (MacLeod et al., 1997). This distorted thinking may activate maladaptive coping behaviours and result in suicidal behaviour. In cognitive behaviour therapy, the therapist aims to help the person identify distorted patterns of thinking and the influence of these on their mood and behaviour, and then focuses on helping the person change the way in which he or she interprets events and experiences.

Cognitive behaviour therapy has been shown to be effective in increasing positive future thinking and decreasing levels of depression (MacLeod *et al.*, 1997). A US treatment study has shown cognitive behaviour therapy to be effective in reducing repetition of deliberate self-harm in attempted suicide patients (Brown *et al.*, 2005). In their review of randomised controlled trials targeting suicide attempters, Hawton and colleagues (1998) highlighted that there had been no trials of cognitive behaviour therapy in adolescents who had self-harmed, although the therapy had been used successfully in adolescent patients with depression (Harrington *et al.*, 1998b). In a large US treatment trial, depressed adolescents aged between 12 and 17 years were allocated randomly to receive one of four treatments, each lasting 12 weeks:

- fluoxetine (10–40mg per day) alone
- cognitive behaviour therapy alone
- cognitive behaviour therapy with fluoxetine
- placebo.

The cognitive behaviour therapy programme was intensive, consisting of 15 one-hour sessions. Depression scores improved most in adolescents treated with cognitive behaviour therapy in combination with fluoxetine; the outcome with this treatment was superior to treatment with either fluoxetine alone or cognitive behaviour therapy alone. Fluoxetine alone was also superior to cognitive behaviour therapy alone. Adolescents in all four groups showed a reduction in suicide ideation by the end of the trial, but those treated with cognitive behaviour therapy plus fluoxetine showed the greatest improvement (March *et al.*, 2004). Developments and problems regarding the use of antidepressants to treat adolescents are discussed later.

Family therapy

As noted already, many adolescents who deliberately self-harm have family problems. Therefore, family therapy may be an appropriate treatment approach. This is especially so in younger adolescents. Family therapy is focused primarily on improving communication and problem-solving within the family. The main aim of treatment is to help the adolescent and their family to resolve the difficulties that led to deliberate self-harm.

Family therapy is also used to help the adolescent learn to deal with future problems without recourse to self-harm (Harrington, 2001). Furthermore, since the episode of deliberate self-harm may affect the equilibrium of the family system, family therapy can help to restore balance.

There is only limited evidence concerning the effectiveness of family therapy with adolescent self-harmers. Harrington and colleagues (1998a) carried out a randomised controlled trial in which the control group received treatment as usual and the experimental group received four home visits during which the adolescents and their family members were encouraged to focus on family communication and problem-solving. No significant differences were found between the two groups in terms of repetition of self-harm. However, parents were more satisfied with the family therapy approach. Also, a subgroup of the adolescents who did not suffer from major (i.e. clinical) depression at entry to the study had less suicidal ideation at follow-up if they received family therapy. Harrington and colleagues (1998a) concluded that brief forms of family intervention are likely to be effective only in subjects without major depression and who show less severe forms of suicidal behaviour.

Dialectical behaviour therapy

A particularly intensive form of cognitive behaviour therapy – dialectical behaviour therapy – has been developed by Linehan and colleagues (1991) in the USA. This treatment was designed for patients with borderline personality disorders, including repeated self-harm. In addition to intensive therapist support, it includes help with recognition of emotional reactions, distancing from emotions, problem-solving and development of interpersonal skills. The results of this approach with adult females have been very promising. Dialectical behaviour therapy has also been investigated in adolescents. An inpatient adolescent unit that adopted dialectical behaviour therapy to treat suicidal adolescents reported fewer behavioural incidents compared with an inpatient unit run on psychodynamically oriented principles (Katz et al., 2004). There is clearly a need for further evaluation of this approach, particularly for adolescents with a history of repeated deliberate self-harm and who can be treated on an outpatient basis.

Group therapy

Treatment in a group setting has been tested in adolescents who have repeatedly self-harmed (Wood et al., 2001). In a pilot study, adolescents who were repeaters of self-harm (at least two episodes of self-harm in the preceding year) were assigned randomly to receive either group therapy plus routine care or routine care alone. A variety of therapy techniques was used in the groups, including cognitive behaviour therapy, problem-solving, dialectical behaviour therapy and psychodynamic group psychotherapy. The treatment focused on relationship problems, school problems, family difficulties and anger management. Initial treatment was in an acute group, and later treatment continued in a long-term group. The adolescents who received group therapy attended a median of eight treatment sessions over six months. At follow-up, adolescents in the group therapy condition had repeated self-harm less, had better school attendance and had lower rates of behavioural disorders than those in the routine care alone condition, but the former did not differ from the latter with regard to levels of depression or scores on a global outcome measure. However, the adolescents in the group therapy condition needed less routine care than the other adolescents. We await the results of large-scale evaluation of this promising approach.

Emergency card provision

There has been interest in the UK in providing emergency access to care by giving deliberate self-harm patients a card that allows them to get immediate access to help at times of crisis. This is important given that repetition of self-harm may occur relatively impulsively. The aim is to prevent crises precipitating repetition of deliberate self-harm. Studies evaluating the provision of an emergency green card given to adult self-harmers have produced mixed results (J. Evans et al.,2005; Evans et al., 1999; Morgan et al., 1993). This approach was also evaluated in a small randomised controlled trial for young adolescents who had presented with deliberate self-harm (Cotgrove et al., 1995). In addition to receiving routine care, adolescents in the experimental group were given an emergency card that allowed them to gain admission to hospital. Those in the control group received routine care alone. Although there was a lower rate of repetition of deliberate self-harm in the emergency card group, the small number of participants in the trial meant that the difference was not statistically significant.

Although it is uncertain whether provision of an emergency card is effective, some clinical services provide selected patients with open telephone access to the service at times of crisis in order to get advice. The usefulness of this strategy for adolescents requires evaluation.

Medication

Because many adolescents who self-harm are suffering from depression, an important question is the extent to which antidepressants are useful in this population. Tricyclic antidepressants do not appear to be effective for adolescents in general with depressive disorders (Keller *et al.*, 2000). In any case, their toxicity in overdose would limit the usefulness in a population clearly at risk of self-poisoning. There is evidence that selective serotonin reuptake inhibitor (SSRI) antidepressants, especially fluoxetine, are effective in the treatment of adolescents with depression. This has received further support from the findings of the Treatment of Adolescent Depression Study (March *et al.*, 2004). However, the use of SSRI antidepressants to treat depression or other disorders in adolescents has received a setback because of the publication of previously unpublished data from trials that suggested that frequency of self-harm and suicidal thoughts may be increased in adolescents receiving SSRIs (except fluoxetine) or the serotonin and noradrenaline reuptake inhibitor (SNRI) venlafaxine (Whittington *et al.*, 2004). This finding prompted guidance from the UK Committee on Safety of Medicines (2004) stating that SSRIs (except fluoxetine) should not be used to treat children and adolescents and a black box warning for these drugs by the US Food and Drug Administration (2004). This has presented some difficulties for clinicians involved in treating depressed adolescents, especially adolescents with a history of self-harm or suicidal ideas. It is likely to result in greater use of psychosocial interventions for such adolescents. This has been reinforced in the guideline from the National Institute for Clinical Excellence (2005) in England, which states that children and adolescents diagnosed with moderate to severe depression should be offered a specific psychological therapy, such as cognitive behavioural therapy, interpersonal therapy or family therapy, as a first line of treatment. When antidepressants are used, this should only be in combination with concurrent psychological therapy, unless the latter is refused. The problem with implementing this guidance is that currently there are insufficient numbers of trained therapists available to provide the amount of therapy that will be required.

Summary and implications

In this chapter, we have highlighted the potential role for the GP in identifying psychosocial problems in adolescents, including those presenting with physical symptoms. It has been suggested that GPs need to make special efforts in order to meet the specific needs of adolescents. A key issue that adolescents have highlighted concerns confidentiality. They may fear that their parents will be involved in their healthcare, which can result in a reluctance to seek help from a GP. There is clearly a need for GP services to give priority to addressing specific problems that adolescents may have in seeking help for emotional problems. We have suggested a possible screening approach to detecting adolescents with difficulties, especially those at risk of self-harm.

Similarly, general hospital emergency departments should include provision of services aimed at young people. This includes ensuring that staff have the skills needed to communicate and deal effectively with challenging young people. In spite of well-established standards published by the Royal College of Psychiatrists (1994, 2004), the management received by individuals who have self-harmed and who present to emergency departments in general hospitals in the UK still varies widely.

The Royal College of Paediatrics and Child Health (2003: pp 47) highlighted that there was 'no formal clinical training in any area of adolescent health in the UK outside of mental health'. There is, therefore, a clear need for training in adolescent health for all healthcare professionals. Given that randomised controlled studies have shown that the necessary skills for helping GPs and other healthcare professionals to deal with young people can be taught and that skills persist over time (Sanci *et al.*, 2000), some training should be included in the undergraduate medical training curriculum as well as at postgraduate levels and during continuing professional development.

All adolescents who present to hospital or in other settings following deliberate self-harm should receive a full psychosocial assessment. We have provided details of how this might be conducted. In terms of subsequent treatment options, we have focused on interventions that aim to target emotional or behavioural disorders and those that aim to prevent the repetition of deliberate self-harm. We have shown that there is no consensus regarding the best therapeutic intervention for adolescents who engage in deliberate self-harm. Few treatment trials have focused specifically on adolescents. In spite of the inconclusive evidence regarding the effectiveness of the different psychotherapeutic approaches, some interventions, such as cognitive behavioural therapy, problem-solving therapy, family therapy and group therapy, may be used in the treatment of individuals who have self-harmed. Finally, because many adolescents who self-harm have symptoms of depression, an important question is the extent to which antidepressants are useful in this population. Although there is evidence that SSRI antidepressants are effective in the treatment of adolescents with depression, some data suggest that the frequency of self-harm and suicidal thoughts may, occasionally, be increased in adolescents receiving SSRIs. This clearly presents problems for clinicians involved in treating depressed adolescents, and is likely to lead to greater use of psychosocial interventions.

In this chapter, we have discussed the role that the health service can play in identifying adolescents at risk of self-harm and managing those who have self-harmed. In the next chapter, we consider alternative sources of support that young people who engage in deliberate self-harm can access. We also highlight the potential influence of media portrayal and reporting of suicidal behaviour on the risk of self-harm in adolescents.

CHAPTER 8

Self-help, Crisis Lines, the Internet and the Media and Deliberate Self-harm

Introduction

In this chapter, we explore alternative sources of support to which adolescents can turn. In particular, we focus on self-help books, telephone help-lines and the Internet. Such resources can be helpful if the young person is not in treatment or does not want treatment. They may help to decrease the young person's sense of being alone and perhaps his or her thinking that he or she is the only one with such problems. This might also fuel a desire to seek treatment. Resources such as self-help and the Internet may also be useful when a young person is on the waiting list for treatment. Child and adolescent mental health services are increasingly using self-help books to assist those who are waiting for treatment. These resources may also be helpful when used in conjunction with treatment, and they may be of value for friends, parents and people who come into contact with, or are concerned about, a young person who engages in deliberate self-harm. Finally, we look at the role that media portrayal and reporting of suicidal behaviour may play in influencing self-harm and suicide and the types of portrayal and reporting that may have particularly negative influences. We also explore the potential for media to have a preventive role.

Self-help books

Many books have been written for people who have engaged in deliberate self-harm and for friends, relatives and health workers who come into contact with people who are self-harmers. Some of these books are written by health professionals (e.g. Schmidt and Davidson, 2004); others are contributed to by people who self-harm (e.g. Arnold and McGill, 1998). The books often take the form of self-help manuals. Many of the books aim to teach users important skills, such as:

- understanding and evaluating self-harm

- keeping safe in a crisis

- dealing with seemingly unsolvable problems

- developing additional coping strategies to reduce the need to self-harm.

The extent to which these skills can be taught solely through reading a book requires systematic research. The potential usefulness of self-help books is likely to be particularly uncertain if the young person is depressed and feels that everything is hopeless and nothing can be done. A further problem is that such methods are likely to be more accessible to and usable by adolescents with higher levels of education. There is, however, some promising research on bibliotherapy for a range of difficulties that adolescents may face. For distressed individuals, perhaps the use of a self-help book in conjunction with therapy may be more appropriate. As we have pointed out, many young people who engage in deliberate self-harm have maladaptive cognitive and problem-solving skills, which may mean that they struggle to implement the suggestions in the books without the help of a trained therapist. Nevertheless, the books are an extremely useful source of information for young people to turn to, including at times of crisis. We have provided a list of self-help books for adolescents with emotional problems in Appendix VII.

Confidential telephone services

Telephone helplines can be a useful source of support. Some helplines offer support regardless of the problem; others provide support and advice only for specific problems. Telephone support is within relatively easy reach for young people. For a young person who has not sought support before, making a telephone call may seem less daunting than going to see someone face-to-face (Hill, 1995). Two major sources of support available in the UK are Samaritans (www.samaritans.org) and ChildLine (www.childline.org.uk).

Samaritans may not refer to itself as a suicide-prevention organisation (it offers 24-hour confidential support to people in emotional distress, including those who have suicidal feelings), but reducing the number of people who take their own lives is very much at the heart of its ethos. In effect, Samaritans is the original telephone helpline, offering support to the vast number of callers who contact it each year. In addition to the telephone service, Samaritans has introduced email and text access to support services. Both forms of communication are thought to be likely to appeal to teenagers. At the time of writing, Samaritans receives more than 450 email messages a day from all over the world. Over half of the people contacting Samaritans in this manner express suicidal feelings (a much higher percentage than those using the telephone). Messages are answered within 24 hours. Samaritans believes that email allows people to gain much benefit from the level of anonymity and confidentiality offered, which enables them to say things openly and express the raw intensity of their feelings. This may be because there is an element of distance with email, which means that the normal rules of conversation and pleasantries often needed in human interaction are not necessary.

ChildLine offers support specifically to children and adolescents who are suffering any kind of problem, including abuse, bullying, difficult relationships and suicidal feelings. Young people who are worried about a friend can also call. Those calling ChildLine will talk to a trained counsellor who can help them to decide what to do or where to go for help next. ChildLine offers a free 24-hour telephone counselling service for children and young people. It has provided a listening ear for millions of children in trouble and danger.

In Chapter 5, we highlighted the responses of adolescents in our schools study to the questions concerning how helping agencies could best help people their age who were experiencing problems. Their attitudes towards such agencies were often less positive than might have been expected. Whether this is a reflection of the fact that young people prefer to turn to friends and family when they need help, or a function of their lack of knowledge about what these services could do for them, is open to further exploration. In particular, the adolescents in our schools study were concerned about issues of confidentiality, e.g. the calls being listed on telephone bills, and the stigma they felt was linked to the act of asking for help. They also wanted agencies to be more relevant and accessible for young people. In addition, other researchers have reported that females were more likely than males to use telephone helplines (De Anda and Smith, 1993). There is clearly a need for those responsible for telephone helplines to do all they can to make them attractive to distressed and suicidal youngsters and to maximise their effectiveness.

The Internet

The Internet has opened up vast opportunities for accessing health information. Internet resources for mental healthcare have multiplied rapidly since 1996. Indeed, networked computers now allow patients to connect with other patients as well as health professionals around the world (Bauerle Bass, 2003). This means that people are now able to access medical information that was, until recently, reserved for academics and health professionals. It enables lay people to gain extensive insights into their own health. According to Ferguson (1998), physicians are now reporting that a third or more of their patients are asking them about health information that they have found on the Internet. Patients are also meeting each other on the Internet, giving each other advice and support. Indeed, seekers of health information can obtain advice from millions of online peers and professionals worldwide at any time of day (Eng, 2001). The Internet allows these information seekers to assess their health risks, consider prevention options, decide on treatment regimes and consult a health professional, all without leaving their homes (Barnes *et al.*, 2003).

The Internet has many hundreds of thousands of sites devoted to the topic 'suicide'. These sites can be categorised into four types (Hawton and Williams, 2002). The first group is concerned with the provision of constructive and useful information aimed at providing greater understanding of the reasons for suicidal behaviour. Other sites provide advice and information for people seeking help with dealing with suicidal thoughts. A third category includes chat rooms and bulletin boards, which enable individuals to engage in discussions with each other. Finally, there are sites that provide instructions on suicide methods – so-called recipe sites – or even encourage suicide, perhaps by pairing up suicidal individuals. There has been much media coverage of suicide pacts via the Internet. Although these appear to have some characteristics that differ from our understanding of more traditional pacts, such as being between people who may never have physically met, the information available is anecdotal and requires further research. Suicide pacts in general account for only a small proportion of all deaths, and the role of cyber-pacts within this proportion also requires further systematic evaluation.

As we have noted already, adolescents in particular have reported a reluctance to use helping agencies for a number of reasons, including fear that their anonymity may be compromised, being afraid that their problems are not sufficiently serious to warrant contacting such an agency, embarrassment, and feeling that the people working for the helping agencies do not have the same life experiences as them and so will not be able to understand their perspective. The attraction of the Internet is that at first glance it apparently addresses all these fears.

Perhaps the most important feature of the Internet is the ability to hide ones identity and thus maintain anonymity (McKenna and Bargh, 1998). Anonymity has a disinhibiting effect (Griffiths, 2002), diminishing the pressure of social desirability and encouraging the exchange of true attitudes and opinions. Likened to the concept of 'strangers on a train' (Bargh *et al.*, 2002), these effects promote self-disclosure because the cost of divulging information is reduced significantly. The effects are thought to be amplified further when discussing sensitive topics – indeed, it is entirely likely that someone who would admit to suicidal thoughts or behaviours, including deliberate self-harm, anonymously would not do so if such an admission would lead to their identification (Safer, 1997b; Shochet and O'Gorman, 1995).

Internet support groups

The rapid growth of Internet access has created new possibilities for people with health concerns to engage in supportive communication with a network of individuals who are all coping with the same issue (Walther and Boyd, 2002). Although face-to-face support groups are popular, there are a number of characteristics that are unique to the realm of the Internet that can make this a more attractive proposition. For example, the ability of computer-mediated communication to transcend geographical and temporal constraints (Wright and Bell, 2003) can be particularly useful for adolescents, who perhaps have to rely on parents for transport. Disclosing health information over the Internet can feel less risky than doing so in a face-to-face context. For example, Wallace (1999) noted that people might want to remain anonymous in order to feel able to ask questions that might reveal what they perceive as their stupidity or to voice their concerns about an issue that they feel is not serious enough for them to contact a helping agency using more traditional means. Also, because there are reduced social status cues in the computer-mediated environment, it can be easier to establish supportive relationships. Finally, Internet support groups can reduce the stigma associated with the illness, behaviour or condition that individuals have. Wright (2000) studied computer-mediated groups for people dealing with health-related issues, such as substance abuse problems and mental illness, and found that the most frequently mentioned advantage of these groups was the perception that there was less stigma attached to the condition by other online support group members due to the anonymity of the medium than in the face-to-face world. This is particularly likely to be so for deliberate self-harm, since often a sense of shame, disgrace or taboo is associated with the act, which can prevent young people from seeking help.

A second important point in favour of Internet sources of help and information is the asynchronous (not in real time) nature of corresponding with other group members. Wright and Bell (2003) highlight that asynchronous communication usually occurs when participants send email messages or use bulletin boards to post messages to others. Although feedback is slower using this method, compared with synchronous (real-time) chat rooms, for example, it can be more convenient because the individual can write and respond at times that suit him or her. Another advantage of asynchronous communication is the ability for more than one person to respond to a message. Everyone who is a member of the group can, potentially, read and respond to the message (Wellman, 1997).

Websites providing advice for young people

A good example of the kind of support that can be provided online has been developed by a GP and a consultant in public health. The aim was to develop two linked websites designed to provide teenagers with 'cringe-free' information in an entertaining way. These websites were set up in February 2000 with the aid of young people, using actual and virtual focus groups. Since their launch, the websites have had over 15 million hits and receive more than 1000 emailed questions to the site's online doctor every month. The sites are free to the user and contain no advertising.

The first site, www.teenagehealthfreak.org, is an online diary of a hypochondrial teenager 'Pete Payne'. Pete updates his diary daily with his worries and traumas, plus those of his family and friends. Pete soon discovers

Dr Ann's site, and his diary often links with it for information on his latest health worry. Pete's diary provides a teenager-friendly relevant health information resource in a humorous format designed to encourage visitors to return and keep up to date with events. The second site, www.doctorann.org, is the virtual surgery of Pete's doctor, Dr Ann. The surgery is full of evidence-based medical information about common teenage health worries. This site provides a more substantial health information resource. It is split into nine key sections: Emergency Room, Not Feeling Well? Drugs and Alcohol, Sex, Smoking, Weight and Eating, Body Changes: Girls, Body Changes: Boys and Moods (including depression, self-harm, anxiety and eating disorders). Further sections include quizzes and surveys, a noticeboard and an A–Z index of the site. In addition, teenagers can email the doctor in confidence with their own health problems via the 'Ask Dr Ann' option. Dr Ann cannot respond to all questions, but new key questions and answers appear daily.

There is evidence that promotion of help-seeking from specific websites may be effective. Adolescents in schools in Australia received a presentation on a website, www.reachout.com.au, which aimed to provide information on a range of difficulties such as bullying, loss, relationship problems and mental health problems, including depression, anxiety and suicide. The aims of the website are to increase young people's access to mental health information and to promote positive help-seeking behaviours and coping skills. Six months after the presentation, the majority of the adolescents knew where they could go for help and who they could talk to. Almost half the adolescents had visited the Reach Out! site and approximately two-thirds said that they would use it if they were having a tough time (Nicholas *et al.*, 2004).

The Internet may be particularly attractive to boys, who are more reluctant than girls to seek help from traditional sources. However, in a survey of high-school students in the USA, Gould and colleagues (2002) found that roughly equal proportions of boys and girls reported seeking help via the Internet.

Risks and problems with the Internet environment

Although online venues may appear private and encourage the disclosure of personal thoughts, they are public domains (Murray and Fisher, 2002), affording little guarantee of absolute confidentiality or anonymity. Thus, the risk of interception by a third party is a possibility that cannot be ignored (Murray and Fisher, 2002; Nosek *et al.*, 2002). In addition, it is difficult to discern which resources on the Web are accurate or appropriate for users (Eng, 2001). Because there is a lack of published regulations concerning the Internet, there is a growing concern that a substantial proportion of health information may be inaccurate, misleading or even fraudulent (Barnes *et al.*, 2003). This is especially pertinent when one considers that nearly one-fifth of adolescents in a survey conducted in the USA reported that they had accessed the Internet in order to seek help for emotional problems (Gould *et al.*, 2002, 2004). The primary source that adolescents turned to for help with their emotional problems was chat rooms. These create the environment whereby people with concerns about a particular issue, such as deliberate self-harm, can engage in communication with a network of other individuals who are all coping with similar problems that are difficult to talk about in a face-to-face environment away from the Internet. However, chat rooms are generally unsupervised and, thus, it is possible that misinformation as well as constructive and supportive advice can be exchanged.

Linked to the issue of the kind of information that can be accessed via the Internet, a further issue of concern revolves around the ability of consumers, and adolescents in particular, to evaluate the quality of the Internet sites and the information that they access. For example, Barnes and colleagues (2003) found that although e-health consumers were generally able to judge the quality of a website, their final assessment of the quality was often influenced by the layout and appeal of the website.

How do adolescents decide on the credibility of a website or chat room? What is it about a website that encourages the user to stop or to go further with their search for information? How can users be certain that the other users offering information are who they say they are? The lack of non-verbal cues through the channel of Internet communication means that deception can be facilitated (Wright and Bell, 2003).

There has been a proliferation of Internet sites that focus on the topic of deliberate self-harm, but not always in a professional and objective manner. Because of the lack of published regulations for the Internet, there is growing concern that these less professional sites may be harmful to an adolescent population and, at the extreme, may actually encourage adolescents to engage in self-harming behaviour, with potentially very serious consequences.

There is also a belief that consumers lack the ability to evaluate the information that they are presented with (Fornaciari and Roca, 1999). As such, it has been argued that educational efforts are required to teach Internet users how to rate and retrieve quality information. This would be a mammoth task. Thus, in line with the conclusions drawn by Gould and colleagues (2002), we believe that attention would be better directed towards raising standards, improving the resources and introducing a way of monitoring and systematically evaluating sites, particularly those aimed at an adolescent population who may not possess the necessary skills to be able to evaluate objectively the information offered to them. Perhaps a system of grading of websites could be introduced and shared with search engines to ensure that those that meet the grading criteria appear more prominently in search results.

The Media

In this section of the chapter, we focus on the role that the media may play in relation to deliberate self-harm and consider the potential role it could have in the prevention of suicidal behaviour. Research in several countries, especially in the UK and the USA, strongly indicates that media representation can and does lead to copycat behaviour (Hawton and Williams, 2002; Pirkis and Blood, 2001). Although there have been several studies that have not shown a media effect, there are many examples of increases in suicide and deliberate self-harm linked to the way in which suicidal behaviour has been portrayed or reported. For example, Phillips (1974) showed that the more publicity a suicide case was given, especially when on the front pages of a newspaper, the more suicides were found in the period following publication. Schmidtke and Häfner (1988) demonstrated a similar effect of a six-episode German television series entitled *Death of a Student*, which showed the railway suicide of a 19-year-old male student. In five of the six episodes, the scene of the suicide was shown at the beginning. After the series, an increase in railway suicides was found over several weeks. This was especially true for the gender and age group that closely resembled the student in the series. Similarly, Hawton and colleagues (1999c) showed that after an episode of the UK hospital drama *Casualty*, which had featured a paracetamol overdose, hospital presentations for self-poisoning increased by 17 per cent in the week following the broadcast and by 9 per cent in the second week. In fact, 20 per cent of the patients who had seen the episode said that it had influenced their decision to take an overdose. There was a specific effect on use of paracetamol for self-poisoning in those who saw the episode and subsequently took an overdose.

Those most affected by the media appear to be young people. The risks seem to be greater when there is a feeling of identification, such as in the case of celebrity death by suicide or the death by suicide of an attractive fictional character. The provision of the details of the methods used for suicidal acts seems to be a particularly potent factor likely to increase the risk of suicidal behaviour.

Preventing media influences on suicidal behaviour

One approach to preventing media reporting and portrayal of suicide having a negative effect on suicidal behaviour in the community is to develop guidelines for the media. To be successful, these must be produced in conjunction with representatives of the media and, thus, be jointly owned.

In their guidelines for the media concerning the portrayal of suicide, Samaritans (2002) accept that suicide is a valid subject for both reporting and dramatic representation, but they make the point that certain types of media coverage are considered to be potentially harmful and can act as a catalyst that could influence the behaviour of those who are already vulnerable. In particular, Samaritans suggest that young people can be most affected by media coverage, particularly when there is a feeling of identification, perhaps in the case of a celebrity death by suicide. They also state that it is dangerous to provide specific details of a suicide method because this can offer a vulnerable person the knowledge that they need in order to carry out an act of deliberate self-harm or suicide.

In a similar vein, Schmidtke and Schaller (2000) have highlighted an association in different countries between how the mass media report suicide and attitudes towards suicide and suicide prevention. The way in which different countries portray suicide in the newspapers hints at differences in the acceptance of suicide. For example, US headlines label suicide in a more criminalising way, but suicide is portrayed more commonly as a tragedy and political protest in Hungarian headlines (Fekete *et al.*, 1998). The portrayal of positive consequences of suicidal behaviour is thought to increase the possibility of identification with suicide and, thus, more imitation. Therefore, a dangerous message from the media is that suicide achieves results – for example, it makes people sorry or it makes them praise the individual who dies.

Since the association between media portrayal and suicidal behaviour appears to be strongest in young people (Hawton and Williams, 2002), improvements in the way in which suicidal behaviour is dealt with by the media may have special relevance to the prevention of self-harm and suicide in the young. For example, suicides on the Viennese subway system were increasing from 1984. The major Austrian newspapers portrayed these deaths in a very sensational and dramatic way. In 1987, the Austrian Association for Suicide Prevention published media guidelines that changed the characteristics of reporting the suicides. Instead of printing sensational stories, the newspapers printed short reports that were rarely on the front page, or did not mention the suicides at all. Sonneck and colleagues (1994) found that the number of suicides on the subway decreased significantly in the second half of 1987, and the rates remained low. A similar successful initiative also involving reporting of subway suicides took place in Toronto (Littman, 1983). Another example demonstrating how important the nature of newspaper coverage is concerns the death of the American singer Kurt Cobain. There was no increase in suicide rates following his death by suicide in his home town Seattle. This was believed to be because the reporting differentiated strongly between the brilliance of his achievements and the wastefulness of his death and also the effect of Courtney Love, his partner, telling people how angry she was with him (Jobes *et al.*, 1996; Kienhorst, 1994). In Switzerland, Michel and colleagues (2000) showed that changes in the nature of newspaper reporting of suicides, with reduced risk of imitation, can be achieved through collaboration with newspaper editors. This initiative did not, however, include evaluation of its impact on suicide rates.

Several organisations have put together guidelines highlighting good practice for the mass media in the reporting and portrayal of suicidal behaviour (e.g. American Foundation for Suicide Prevention, American Association of Suicidology and Annenberg Public Policy Center, 2001; MediaWise Trust, 2003; Samaritans, 2002). To be effective locally, it is clear that such guidelines must be developed in full collaboration with the media representatives in the country. A summary of the key points made by these guidelines suggests that the following are needed in the reporting of suicidal phenomena:

- There should be limiting of the dramatic or sensational coverage given to suicides: stories should not be reported on the front pages of newspapers and no photographs should be included.

- Reports should avoid explicit details of the method, such as the drug taken or the number of tablets taken in overdoses. Reporting that a person died from carbon monoxide poisoning, for example, is probably not in itself harmful, but providing details of the mechanism and procedure used to carry out the suicide may lead to imitation of suicidal behaviour by other people at risk.

- The issue needs to be explained in a sensitive manner, with the aim of educating the public.

- Reports should avoid presenting the message that suicide achieves results. For example, reporting that highlights community expressions of grief may suggest that the local community is honouring the suicidal behaviour of the deceased person rather than mourning their death.

- There should be an avoidance of the use of simplistic explanations for suicide. Suicide is rarely the result of a single factor (although a catalyst for the behaviour might seem to be obvious) and is often linked with mental health illnesses/conditions, such as depression.

- Suicide should never be portrayed as an understandable way of problem-solving. Where appropriate, the contact details of helping agencies such as Samaritans should be presented alongside the media item in question.

One further aspect of potential prevention of suicidal behaviour through the media is that of modelling positive coping and help-seeking strategies when young people are faced by crises of the kind that may result in suicidal acts. In this manner, the media, especially television, have enormous potential power to contribute to the prevention of suicidal behaviour. For example, inclusion of such initiatives in television soap operas popular with teenagers could be very effective. A positive collaboration between media producers and experts in prevention in this regard would be a very fruitful way forward. Of course, any such initiatives of this kind should be evaluated carefully.

Summary and implications

In this chapter, we have explored alternative sources of support to which adolescents can turn. A widely available source of support is self-help books, many of which aim to teach users important skills. However, as we have highlighted, many young people who engage in deliberate self-harm have maladaptive cognitive and problem-solving skills, which may mean that they have difficulty implementing the suggestions without the support and guidance of a trained therapist. Nevertheless, we believe that self-help books are a useful resource, not least because they provide adolescents with an accessible source of information to which they might turn at times of difficulty.

Another accessible source of support is confidential telephone helplines. We highlighted the services offered by Samaritans and ChildLine that young people can access as an instant means of gaining support when they are thinking about or have actually engaged in forms of suicidal behaviour. In Chapter 5, we highlighted some of the attitudes held by the adolescents who took part in our schools study about helping agencies in general. In particular, adolescents expressed concerns about issues of confidentiality and the stigma that they feel surrounds the act of asking for help. This raises questions as to how such agencies can better advertise their services so that adolescents realise just what is available to them and how they can access such services in a confidential manner.

The Internet is a form of self-help that has opened up vast opportunities for accessing health information. Perhaps the most important feature of the Internet is the ability to hide one's identity and thus maintain anonymity, both being issues to which adolescents attach great importance. We highlighted the very successful Teenage Health Freak website, which provides help and advice to adolescents with health concerns.

However, in spite of the many positive benefits associated with the Internet, there are concerns that the quality of some of the sites may be low and that some may be harmful. It is, therefore, important to explore how adolescents decide on the credibility of particular websites and chat rooms. Attention should be directed towards raising standards, improving resources and introducing a method of monitoring and evaluating sites, particularly those aimed at the adolescent population. Some countries, e.g. Denmark, have moved towards regulating suicide recipe sites provided through national Internet site providers, although the nature of the Internet makes this a challenging task.

Finally, we focused on the role of the media in relation to suicidal behaviour. Research from the UK, the USA and other countries strongly indicates that media representation can and does lead to copycat behaviour. We have shown that those most affected by the influence of the media also appear to be young people. We have suggested how the power of the media can be harnessed and used positively as a tool to help with prevention of suicidal behaviour. We call for responsible media reporting and portrayal of suicide and have highlighted guidelines for good practice.

In the next and final chapter, we draw together and summarise the main points and conclusions discussed in this book. We also highlight important future needs in this field.

CHAPTER 9

Conclusions and Looking to the Future

This book is about the problem of deliberate self-harm in adolescents. Self-harming behaviour is one of the key health problems in this age group. As we have shown, it is symptomatic of a wide range of factors. Our own community-based study of deliberate self-harm in adolescents in schools has been central to the book. In addition, we have drawn from the international literature to set our findings in context and to provide a more comprehensive picture of the problem of deliberate self-harm in adolescents. In this chapter, we summarise the main points and findings covered in the book. We then highlight their implications for clinical practice, prevention initiatives, research and society in general.

In Chapter 2, we indicated how the type of approach used in surveys of sensitive information in adolescents is crucial in determining the validity of the results that are obtained. We then described the careful methodology that we used in our schools study. We believe that the approach that we used, although not perfect, addressed many of the limitations of other research investigations of this kind.

In Chapter 3, we described our initial results in terms of the extent of the problem of deliberate self-harm among adolescents who took part in our schools study. Overall, 6.9 per cent of the adolescents reported and described an episode of deliberate self-harm in the preceding year that met our study criteria. One in 10 had engaged in deliberate self-harm at some time during their young lives. A further 15 per cent of the adolescents reported having had thoughts about harming themselves in the previous year but had not gone on to do so. The extent of these phenomena in adolescents in our study highlights the size of the problem of deliberate self-harm and thoughts of self-harm in adolescents. The findings from our study are not unusual. We have shown from our review of the international literature (Evans *et al.*, 2005a) that the rates of self-harm and thoughts of self-harm in our study are very much in keeping with those found in investigations conducted elsewhere, particularly in the USA. Furthermore, the prevalence of self-harm in our study is similar to that found in some other countries in Europe (Ireland, Belgium, Norway) and in Australia, which were part of a collaborative study that used exactly the same methodology as that employed in our schools study. However, lower rates of deliberate self-harm were found in the Netherlands and Hungary.

Until now, most studies of deliberate self-harm in adolescents have been based on adolescents who present to hospitals. This is understandable, since the main clinical response to adolescents who self-harm will be focused on those who come to clinical attention. However, the results of our schools study have shown that adolescents seen at hospital after deliberate self-harm represent an atypical sample of the overall population of adolescents who self-harm at the community level. This is particularly true for the different methods of self-harm. By far the most common method of deliberate self-harm in the adolescents in our schools study was self-cutting. However, the vast majority of adolescents who present to hospitals following deliberate self-harm have taken overdoses. This was confirmed in our study, in which we showed that overdose was the principal distinguishing characteristic of those self-harmers who presented to hospital. However, it should also be noted that more than three-quarters of the adolescents in our study who reported taking overdoses in the preceding year did not present to hospital. This is a surprising and worrying finding, especially since many of the overdoses reported by these adolescents included relatively dangerous substances, especially paracetamol. These findings also show that if there was a small shift in the proportion of adolescents at the community level taking overdoses, then this could have a marked effect on rates based on hospital presentations. For example, the annual rate of deliberate self-harm in our study at the community level was 5875 per 100,000, but the rate based on those who presented to hospital was 840 per 100,000, a figure very similar to that found in hospital-based studies (Hawton *et al.*, submitted). Since most of those presenting to hospital had taken overdoses, a small shift in this proportion at the community level could result in either a significant rise or a major reduction in hospital presentations, depending on the direction of the change. This could have a considerable effect on clinical services, especially if the numbers were to rise. This possibility also needs to be borne in mind when interpreting secular trends based on hospital presentations.

Deliberate self-harm in our schools study was nearly four times more frequent in the girls than the boys. From our review of the international literature (Evans *et al.*, 2005a) this ratio is clearly consistent with findings from elsewhere. Thus, compared with boys, girls are much more likely to report deliberate self-harm or suicide attempts, and to have thoughts of self-harm. This finding is also compatible with those of studies that rely on data obtained from hospital presentations, in which the average rate of deliberate self-harm in adolescents is consistently higher in girls (e.g. Hawton *et al.*, 2003b; Lewinsohn *et al.*, 2001; O'Loughlin and Sherwood, 2005). Also, we have shown from our hospital-based register of deliberate self-harm presentations in Oxford that the female/male ratio is greatest in very young adolescents and then diminishes to approximately two to one in the late teens (Hawton *et al.*, 2003b).

There has been much debate about why there should be such a difference in the rates of deliberate self-harm and thoughts of self-harm between the two sexes, particularly in the teenage years, especially when rates of actual suicide are far higher in males than females. Likely reasons include the earlier experience of puberty in girls and the possible consequences of this for mood disturbances; the tendency of girls to get involved in serious relationships earlier than boys, with consequent distress when such relationships break up; girls having higher rates of mood disorder than boys; and boys more often using other outlets for expression of distress, such as delinquent acts and aggression.

Investigation of the motives for deliberate self-harm in our schools study indicated that the most frequent motive was that the behaviour was a means of coping with distress. Other motives reflected the interpersonal nature of difficulties experienced by many of the adolescents. These findings are in keeping with those from hospital-based studies (e.g. Hawton *et al.*, 1982a). However, many of the adolescents who had engaged in deliberate self-harm indicated that they had wished to die. It is unclear to what extent this reflects a true intention to die or a young person feeling so bad that they feel as if they want to die without really wishing to end up dead. Further research is required in order to clarify the extent to which these two aspects of the to-die motive apply. This might include in-depth interviews of adolescents who have self-harmed.

Self-cutting was the most frequent method of self-harm in our schools study. Very little attention has been paid to the motives involved in self-cutting in adolescents compared with those involved in overdoses. We compared the adolescents who had cut themselves with those who had taken overdoses. More of those who had taken overdoses indicated that they had wanted to die. This was found in both the spontaneous responses to an open-ended question and also the adolescents' choices from the list of eight motives they were shown when asked to select those that applied to them. Self-cutting is often associated with tension reduction and self-punishment, which was reported by many of the girls who cut themselves in our study. This has also been found in studies of clinical samples of females who have cut themselves (e.g. Hawton, 1990; Shearer, 1994). It is clearly relevant to prevention and treatment of self-cutting, in terms of both whether other methods of tension reduction can be encouraged and the need to address the self-esteem issues that may underlie self-cutting.

It has become increasingly obvious from studies such as ours that quite a lot of boys cut themselves. Data based on hospital presentations have shown that increasing numbers of males in general are presenting following self-cutting (Hawton *et al.*, 2004a; Horrocks *et al.*, 2003). We know far less about self-cutting in boys than girls. There is a need for investigation of boys who use this method of deliberate self-harm, particularly to understand the problems they face and the motives behind the self-harm. Certainly the results of our schools study suggest that there are differences in the motivation for self-cutting between male and female adolescents. This may have relevance to both prevention and treatment of self-cutting in young males.

We have shown that deliberate self-harm in adolescents is often highly impulsive, in the sense of the act being carried out with relatively little forethought. Thus, in our schools study, almost half of those who cut themselves and over a third of those who took overdoses said that they had thought about harming themselves for less than an hour beforehand. This does not mean that there had not been prior thinking about self-harm – indeed, we believe that the process leading up to self-harm is often protracted and can be traced over days, weeks, months or, in some cases, even years (Runeson *et al.*, 1996; Van Heeringen, 2001). However, the immediate psychological processes that lead to self-harm are likely to be very rapid. This means that there is often little time for intervention once thoughts of self-harm have been formulated fully. Although efforts to encourage adolescents to seek help at such times are important – and this is a specific time when telephone helplines and seeking help from friends, family and clinical services are very relevant – prevention should be focused mainly on reducing the problems that lead to thoughts of self-harm and helping young people to acquire alternative methods of problem-solving and recognising sources of help. We believe that one of the main approaches to this should be through educational programmes in mental health awareness in schools as well as education via the media. This is discussed further later in this chapter.

We have confirmed that repetition of self-harm by adolescents is common. This was already known from studies of hospital samples of adolescents presenting following self-harm, with just over a third in the study in Oxford reporting that they had harmed themselves previously (Hawton *et al.*, 2003b). In our schools study, the extent of repetition was even greater: more than half of the adolescents who had self-harmed reported a previous episode of deliberate self-harm, this proportion being similar for boys and girls. This is important, because repetition of self-harm indicates persistent or recurrent distress. It is also associated in adults with even greater future risk of completed suicide than single episodes of self-harm (Zahl and Hawton, 2004). Clearly, attention needs to be paid to preventing repetition of deliberate self-harm in adolescents. This must be a major focus of treatment for self-harmers who have been identified through clinical services. It is less clear how one might prevent repetition in those who do not present to services, but educational programmes and self-help approaches represent potentially relevant measures.

A fair amount of attention has been paid to the impact of suicide on relatives and friends. We reviewed studies that have shown that depression is common in mothers (especially) and siblings of adolescents who have died by suicide, and that there are often long-term consequences in terms of psychiatric disorders in relatives. However, far less attention has been paid to the effects that deliberate self-harm and attempted suicide in adolescents may have on other people. Indeed, we are aware of only one study of significance in this field. This showed that mothers experienced a wide range of reactions, including anxiety, guilt, sadness and hostility, and that some of their reactions varied according to whether the deliberate self-harm act was a first episode or a repeat. Fathers, few of whom were included in the study, also reported varied reactions but felt that especially following the deliberate self-harm episode they had to be very careful what they said to their son or daughter (Wagner *et al.*, 2000). This much-neglected aspect of deliberate self-harm in adolescents (and indeed adults) needs more attention. Anecdotal evidence indicates that the impact of having a son or daughter carry out an act of self-harm can be devastating and can have major effects on other family members and friends. Not only does their distress require attention in its own right, but also their reactions to the act are likely to be very significant for subsequent therapy and outcome (King *et al.*, 1997). This is, therefore, an important area for further research. The impact of the behaviour on other people and their response to the adolescent needs to be considered carefully and addressed by clinicians and other helpers dealing with adolescents who have self-harmed.

One important aspect of the reaction of other people to deliberate self-harm is their understanding of the motives involved. If this differs from that of the adolescent, then potentially this can have important consequences. Certainly such differences have been demonstrated between adolescents who have presented to hospital following overdoses and the clinicians who have assessed them (Hawton *et al.*, 1982a). Similar differences in attribution of motives have been found between adults who have taken overdoses and their relatives (James and Hawton, 1985). In therapeutic work with adolescents (and adults) and their families, this needs to be addressed because such differences may cause misunderstandings and undermine treatment. It was a feature of the family problem-solving therapy approach utilised by Harrington and colleagues (1998a) for adolescents who had self-harmed and their families.

The findings from our schools study and from other studies in this area regarding motives for overdoses and self-injury highlight the need for clinicians to explore motives for self-harm. Through understanding the motivation for the behaviour, not only will the clinician obtain a fuller picture of the nature of self-harm in individual cases but also this may help them to decide which strategies may be useful for preventing further episodes of self-harm. Thus, if specific motives can be identified, then the clinician can work with the adolescent to try to develop coping strategies that can be used in the future if the adolescent is confronted by similar circumstances to those that previously preceded previous self-harm.

In Chapter 4, we went on to examine in detail the specific factors that are associated with deliberate self-harm and thoughts of self-harm in adolescents. We did this by considering the results from our schools study and those from other studies reported in the international literature (Evans *et al.*, 2004). We have commented above on gender differences in this behaviour. Much attention has been paid to the frequency of deliberate self-harm in different ethnic groups. In the UK most attention regarding ethnicity and suicidal behaviour has been paid to Asian females, with some studies suggesting that they are at increased risk for self-harm and suicide compared with other females. However, in our schools study, we found that Asian girls were significantly less likely to report self-harm than were white females (Hawton *et al.*, 2002). The findings of a study from London have suggested that adolescent Asian girls are at no more risk of self-harm than other females (Bhugra *et al.*, 2003). An important aspect of the impact of ethnicity on risk of self-harm and suicide is the relative size of a particular ethnic group in a locality in relation to other ethnic groups. Thus, where an ethnic group represents the majority of the population locally, then suicide rates are unlikely to be elevated in that group, whereas where an ethnic group is in the minority, increased rates of suicidal behaviour may be found in that group (Neeleman and Wessely, 1999). This may well be related to the social pressures of being in a minority group, including the possible impact of prejudice and marginalisation. Thus, in interpreting the results of studies of suicidal behaviour in different ethnic groups, the context of such studies needs to be borne in mind. The majority of the Asian adolescents in our schools study were in schools in Birmingham, which has a large Asian population. Thus, it is perhaps not surprising that the rates of deliberate self-harm reported were not elevated compared with those in white pupils.

Both our schools study and other studies in this field have examined a wide range of psychosocial and health factors that might distinguish adolescents who engage in deliberate self-harm from other adolescents and also those who have thoughts of self-harm from other adolescents. There is a consistent finding that depression and anxiety are associated with deliberate self-harm, although the results of our study suggest that the association is stronger in females. We also found that low self-esteem was an important risk factor for deliberate self-harm in both boys and girls. Impulsivity seemed to be a risk factor just in females. This latter finding may be due to the fact that our ability to examine associations between psychological characteristics and deliberate self-harm was greater in the girls because of the larger number of female than male self-harmers. There is good evidence that many adolescents are not very aware of mental health issues (Fortune *et al.*, Heled and Read, 2005; submitted). This is perhaps surprising given the increasing attention to such issues in the media. It again highlights the need for mental health awareness programmes in schools to help young people recognise and understand psychological distress, both in themselves and in their peers.

Such programmes clearly need to include a focus on how adolescents can get help, whether for themselves or for their friends.

Both alcohol and drug use are clearly associated with deliberate self-harm. In our schools study, drug use was one of the strongest predictors of deliberate self-harm for both males and females. The results of other studies support this finding. Other studies also indicate that the association is considerably stronger for hard drugs such as cocaine and heroin than for softer drugs such as cannabis. This is understandable in the sense that cannabis is used so widely that it would be surprising if it was a particularly strong risk factor. For alcohol, although there appears to be an incremental effect of the amount of alcohol consumed, our results suggest that the link with deliberate self-harm may not be direct but may be mediated by other factors, such as depression, anxiety and the effects of alcohol on impulsivity. Nevertheless, school-based and other programmes aimed at the prevention of alcohol and drug abuse are likely to be extremely important in terms of prevention of self-harm and suicidal behaviour among adolescents.

In our schools study, there was also an association between deliberate self-harm and smoking, a finding that is again in agreement with those of other studies (reviewed by Evans *et al.*, 2004). The relationship between smoking and deliberate self-harm is, however, likely to be mediated by other factors.

Problems within families are clearly extremely important in the aetiology of deliberate self-harm. This is a consistent finding across studies in this field. A specific association has been found with sexual and physical abuse (Evans *et al.*, 2004). Ongoing discord within families, break-up of parental marriages, mental health issues and alcohol abuse are also linked strongly to the risk of deliberate self-harm in adolescents. This highlights the importance of any initiatives to reduce family dysfunction and the potential need for family therapy for some adolescents who present with deliberate self-harm.

Peer relationships are also extremely important. Having difficulty keeping friends and having arguments with friends are associated significantly with increased risk of deliberate self-harm and thoughts of self-harm. Further important issues concern schoolwork, including difficulties with keeping up with schoolwork and perceived or real academic pressure.

Bullying is clearly an extremely important risk factor for self-harm and suicidal behaviour in adolescents. We found this in our schools study, although other factors tended to outweigh the impact of bullying when we conducted a multivariate statistical analysis. This does not mean, however, that bullying is a minor factor. Indeed, several studies now point to its importance in relation to risk of deliberate self-harm (Kaltiala-Heino *et al.*, 1999; Rigby and Slee, 1999). Clearly, bullying and other abuse (physical as well as sexual) are likely to have major effects on self-esteem and, hence, on mood and vulnerability to thoughts of self-harm in adolescents.

Increasing evidence points to the potential role of sexual orientation difficulties in relation to the risk of deliberate self-harm in adolescents and young adults (Catalan, 2000; Wagman Borowsky *et al.*, 1999). In our schools study, we also found that concerns about sexual orientation were associated with risk of deliberate self-harm, although the association did not appear to be a direct one, perhaps because of the relatively low rate of reporting of such concerns. Interestingly, a study of young people has suggested that the risk of deliberate self-harm may be particularly high in those where there is mixed sexual orientation – that is, where individuals have both heterosexual and homosexual interests (Fergusson *et al.*, 2005a). Presumably, however, the risk of suicidal behaviour in young people with sexual orientation concerns is likely to decrease gradually as variations in sexual orientation become more socially accepted. Nevertheless, there is clearly a need to recognise the impact that such concerns can have on young people, and awareness of this needs to be incorporated in school-based sexual health programmes.

It has become increasingly apparent that exposure to deliberate self-harm by others can be a major risk factor for deliberate self-harm. In our schools study, having a friend who had self-harmed recently was one of the strongest risk factors for deliberate self-harm in both girls and boys. This applied principally to self-cutting and was most marked in females. The finding concerning the general importance of exposure to self-harm is consistent with those of several previous studies (e.g. Bjarnason and Thorlindsson, 1994; Wagman Borowsky *et al.*, 1999). This is important to bear in mind in relation to how schools deal with self-harm. The guidelines for school staff included in Appendix III may be useful in this respect. This finding should also be borne in mind by clinicians when assessing adolescents who have self-harmed or are thought to be at risk of this behaviour. This association is also relevant to educational programmes in schools aimed at preventing risk of self-harm.

In Chapter 4, we also discussed the potential mechanisms that may underlie the important influence that media reporting and portrayal of suicidal behaviour and self-harm can have on the risk of self-harm, although we did not investigate this specifically in our schools study.

In Chapter 5, we highlighted two aspects of adolescents' behaviour relevant to managing difficult situations. The first of these aspects is the extent to which adolescents who are in difficulties perceive themselves as having problems and to be in need of help. It is important to recognise that many troubled adolescents do not view themselves as having problems. This was the case for a quarter of the adolescents in our schools study who had carried out acts of deliberate self-harm. Results of studies in other countries have been consistent with this finding. This suggests that one aspect of pre-vention of deliberate self-harm may involve helping adolescents to recognise when they have problems, how to identify what the problems are and how severe they may be.

Help-seeking behaviour is another important aspect of managing diffi-cult situations. One crucial component of help-seeking is communication with others. In our schools study, adolescents who had carried out acts of deliberate self-harm and those with thoughts of self-harm indicated fewer categories of people with whom they felt able to talk about things that really bothered them than did other adolescents. A particularly worrying finding from our schools study was that of those with a history of a recent deliberate self-harm episode, 20 per cent reported that no one knew about it. Also, 40 per cent of the adolescents who reported having experienced thoughts of self-harm had not talked about them or tried to get help from anyone. One possibility is that when certain adolescents develop problems, they tend to isolate themselves from potential sources of support. Another possibility is that it is the lack of support that contributes to the development of suicidal phenomena. A further possible explanation is that adolescents with problems tend to have fewer people to whom they can turn because the nature of their problems has alienated potential sources of support. These possibilities merit further investigation. In our schools study, we looked at the factors that appeared to get in the way of adolescents seeking help before deliberate self-harm. A few indicated that they did not seek help because they wanted to die. However, the most common responses were that the ado-lescents had felt that they did not need or did not want help. Some explained that they thought that their problems were not serious enough for them to seek help. Others acknowledged that they had problems but thought that they should be able to deal with them themselves. In addition, some adoles-cents had clearly felt shame about their problems or behaviour or had feared how others might react to their problems. Furthermore, some thought that other people would not understand their behaviour or that no one would be able or want to help them.

When the adolescents in our schools study were asked about the people with whom they felt they could talk about things that bothered them, the vast majority indicated their friends as being the main people they turned to. Similarly, those adolescents who had recently deliberately harmed themselves and sought help beforehand had most often turned to their friends rather than other people. Furthermore, friends were the people most likely to know about a deliberate self-harm episode and to attempt to provide help afterwards. Adolescents with thoughts of self-harm also indicated that they were most likely to seek help from their peers. These findings, which are consistent with those of other studies, are extremely important. They indicate the potential burden that adolescents face in terms of supporting their peers. However, most adolescents have not been coached in any way in how best to do this. Therefore, attention to this aspect of support for adolescents should be an essential part of mental health education in schools. In addition to helping adolescents see what they can do to help others, it is essential that they are also given advice on when they should seek help from an adult for a peer in distress because of concerns about the risk to their friend. This may, of course, involve breaching confidentiality. They need help in seeing how this might, in the long term, be the most helpful way of assisting a very troubled friend and keeping them safe.

Parents are another important potential source of support. In our schools study, approximately two-thirds of adolescents said that they would turn to their mother for help. Parents can get advice on how to help troubled adolescents. Some of the self-help material suggested in Appendix VII of this book may be useful in this respect. Teachers were viewed relatively rarely as a source of help by adolescents in our schools study. This is perhaps understandable, since pupils may be afraid that if they confide in a teacher what they say may not remain confidential. They might also see this as conflicting with other roles that the teacher has. Nevertheless, teachers would also benefit from help and advice on how best to identify and support pupils who may be at risk or who have engaged in deliberate self-harm. This may require the help of other agencies that they can to turn to for support. The guidelines for school staff in Appendix III might be helpful in this respect. Another possibility, which was suggested by quite a lot of pupils in our study, is that there should be designated individuals within the school who do not necessarily have a teaching role but who are clearly there to provide confidential advice and support. This already happens in some schools and merits serious consideration. Choice of the most appropriate person must reflect both their skills and his or her being the sort of person that troubled adolescents will approach.

We found important differences between the adolescents in our study who had engaged in deliberate self-harm or had had thoughts of self-harm compared with other adolescents in their reported use of coping strategies. Thus, they tended more often to indicate that they used emotion-focused coping strategies, such as getting angry or having an alcoholic drink, when faced with problems. In addition, they were less likely to employ strategies that actively focused on their problems, such as talking to someone or trying to sort things out. This is in keeping with other studies, which indicate that adolescents who deliberately self-harm may have difficulties with problem-solving (reviewed by Speckens and Hawton, 2005). As a result of these difficulties, such adolescents are less able to cope effectively with problems in their lives, which would also increase their risk of repeat episodes of deliberate self-harm. Depression is a specific factor that seems to undermine problem-solving and increases the risk of repetition of self-harm (Hawton *et al.*, 1999b; Kingsbury *et al.*, 1999).

In Chapter 6, we turned to the potential for prevention of suicidal behaviour through initiatives in schools. We discussed this from three points of view. The first concerned primary prevention, namely efforts to alter factors that might predispose adolescents to thoughts or acts of deliberate self-harm. Some such initiatives have focused specifically on suicide through the provision of suicide-awareness programmes. However, the results of these programmes have been inconsistent, and there are concerns that they can have negative consequences for adolescents. For example, it is possible that they may encourage some adolescents to view suicide as a legitimate response to stress.

As a result of the concerns about educational programmes focused on suicidal behaviour, and because of the recognition that deliberate self-harm and thoughts of self-harm are very often related to psychological and mental health problems, there has been much more focus on the introduction of mental health awareness programmes in schools. This approach is supported further by findings such as the lack of recognition by adolescents that mental health problems can be important contributory factors leading to deliberate self-harm. The content of such programmes might, therefore, include provision of simple information about mental health problems, especially depression and anxiety, and how to recognise them in oneself and in others; training in problem-solving skills; understanding of self-esteem and how this may influence feelings and behaviour and simple strategies for countering negative self-esteem; strategies for coping with stress; where and how to seek help; and how to help others in distress. Unfortunately, evaluation of such programmes has not been very positive to date. The most encouraging results are where such programmes are provided over a lengthy period and where a whole-school approach is used, i.e. where an effort is made to involve everyone associated with the school, including pupils, staff, families and the community, as well as trying to change the environment and culture of the school (reviewed by Wells *et al.*, 2003). It is very important that further development and evaluation of such approaches is carried out in order to determine which approaches are most effective. Evaluations will need to be conducted on a very large scale in order to investigate a range of outcomes and to be sure to identify any negative impacts.

The second broad school-based approach is secondary prevention, which includes efforts to identify adolescents at risk, either because they are experiencing thoughts of self-harm or suicide or because they have characteristics known to be associated with this behaviour. Screening programmes have been investigated, particularly in the USA (Shaffer *et al.*, 2004). This usually involves school pupils initially completing a questionnaire about mood, substance use and suicidal ideation and behaviour. Those who score above a cut-off point are then interviewed to determine whether they have significant problems and whether they require treatment or further evaluation. While there have been some initial encouraging reports of such an approach, there also appear to be major drawbacks. One is that there may be quite a few false-positive cases identified, which will not only be expensive but also risk stigmatisation of the adolescents concerned. Another is that adolescents at risk may not be picked up through this approach, especially those who have fluctuating symptoms. As a result of this, some people have suggested that it is better to train teachers to identify signs that might indicate that pupils are at risk, who can then be referred on to a counsellor.

The third broad preventive approach in schools concerns tertiary prevention, which involves means of dealing with deliberate self-harm or suicide once they have occurred. This is important not only because of the distress that these may cause for peers but also because of the risk of modelling of self-harm and suicide, leading to possible clusters of this behaviour. It is important for schools to have a plan of how they will deal with such situations (e.g. Hazell, 1991). They may need help and advice from outside organisations on how best to manage the situation. The guidelines for school staff in Appendix III might be useful in this respect.

While clearly the main task of schools is the education of pupils, they also undoubtedly have a major potential role in the prevention of deliberate self-harm and suicide. It is clearly important that maximum use is made of the potential of the school environment in this regard. This is certainly an area for further development and evaluation.

In Chapter 7, we focused on the role of the health service in relation to the prevention and management of deliberate self-harm. We began by considering the problems that adolescents appear to have in seeking help from healthcare agencies. Concerns about confidentiality appear to be a major factor. Also, unfamiliarity with accessing such sources of help may be another. In addition, lack of immediacy of access may be a further problem.

General practitioners clearly have a substantial potential role in identifying and helping adolescents who are in difficulty. We have highlighted that this may necessitate awareness that initial presenting symptoms might be misleading, particularly when they are of a physical nature, and, therefore, the need for GPs to be prepared to ask adolescents broad questions about how they are getting on, even if they have presented with apparently innocuous complaints, at least in mental health terms. We have also highlighted the need for general practices to be user-friendly for adolescents and for staff to recognise the difficulties that adolescents may have in approaching their doctors for help. We have outlined a possible screening approach for use in primary care to detect those adolescents with difficulties, and especially those at risk of self-harm. We have also considered approaches to management, including when to refer an adolescent for specialist care. Clearly, primary care should be a major focus for preventive initiatives, and there is a lot that can be done to improve the attractiveness of this potential source of help to adolescents. It is essential that GPs and other primary care staff are educated and trained in the recognition of psychological and mental health problems in adolescents and their management.

In the context of the treatment, we have highlighted the recent problem that has arisen concerning the use of antidepressants in adolescents. This is because examination of published and unpublished data from randomised control trials of SSRI antidepressants has suggested that such drugs may have negative side effects in some adolescents, including the possible development of suicidal ideas and behaviour (Whittington *et al.*, 2004). Legislative authorities have decided that the cost/benefit ratio for these antidepressants is too high, except in the case of fluoxetine, and have recommended that clinicians avoid using them for children and adolescents (UK Committee on Safety of Medicines, 2004; US Food and Drug Administration, 2004). This clearly presents problems for GPs and other clinicians who are trying to manage depression in adolescents. One positive effect of this development might, however, be that there will be more attention to the development and provision of psychological therapies.

We went on to examine the management of adolescents who have engaged in deliberate self-harm and who present to emergency departments in general hospitals. It is accepted that a careful assessment of all such adolescents is essential. We have provided details of an approach to assessment, which we hope will be useful for clinicians. Although knowledge of how to conduct such an assessment is clearly essential, there are other skills that will be very important for ensuring that adolescents get maximum benefits from their hospital attendance. These include attention to attitudes towards adolescents who self-harm, several studies having shown that attitudes of general hospital staff are often negative (Hopkins, 2002; Wilson, 2003). Also, skills are needed in communicating with adolescents with difficulties, especially where they might feel ashamed about the nature of their problems or think that adults will disapprove of them or otherwise not understand them.

The aftercare of adolescents who have presented to hospital with deliberate self-harm is receiving increasing attention. At present, there are no well-established treatment approaches that have been proven to be particularly effective. However, there are strong indications that a psychological approach involving problem-solving and other aspects of cognitive therapy can be effective. Also, a group-therapy approach for adolescents with repetitive self-harm has produced promising results. For some adolescents, family therapy using a problem-solving approach and provided in the adolescents' homes may be helpful (Harrington *et al.*, 1998a).

There are uncertainties about the use of medication in aftercare, although for major psychiatric disorders appropriate physical treatment should be provided. A recent clinical trial comparing cognitive therapy with the use of the SSRI antidepressant fluoxetine in depressed adolescents has suggested that both may be effective, with the combination of fluoxetine and cognitive therapy being particularly potent, especially for reducing suicidal thoughts (March *et al.*, 2004).

In Chapter 8, we explored other sources of support to which adolescents can turn. We considered the role of self-help books and other sources of information that adolescents might find helpful. Although the efficacy of such sources of help for adolescents is uncertain in relation to deliberate self-harm, there are some encouraging signs that they can be helpful for other psychological conditions and problems of adolescents. A crucial question is to what extent will adolescents use self-help resources when in a distressed state? Self-help books may be a useful resource alongside treatment or while adolescents are waiting for treatment. Internet sites may be another source of help. They may be particularly attractive for adolescents who wish to hide their identity or have difficulty communicating directly with others.

Telephone helplines are another important potential source of help. We have particularly highlighted services offered by Samaritans (including email counselling) and ChildLine. Investigations of attitudes held by adolescents towards such sources of help indicate that the sources need to be extremely adolescent-friendly for them to use them. Also, adolescents need to be sure about the confidentiality of any interactions and must overcome any stigma they feel about asking for such help. Thus, the way in which agencies advertise their services is crucial in determining how much they are used and how effective they might be for adolescents.

We also considered the potential dangers of the Internet, especially the safety of certain websites and chat rooms. Of specific concern is that some websites appear to be aimed at encouraging suicidal behaviour. This is particularly true of 'recipe' sites that describe specific methods of suicidal behaviour. Attention needs to be paid to possible legislation to restrict such websites, although this is clearly difficult because of the international nature of the Internet.

Increasingly, it has become clear that the media may play a significant potential role in relation to self-harm and suicide by adolescents. It is now generally accepted that certain types of media portrayal and reporting of suicidal behaviour can encourage such behaviour in viewers and readers. This is particularly so where specific methods of suicide are described or portrayed in detail. Other factors, such as the status or attractiveness to the viewer of a role model who engages in suicidal behaviour, or their similarity to the viewer, may also be important. Because of these findings, guidelines for media portrayal and reporting of suicidal behaviour have been drawn up. There are still problems concerning how acceptable these are to people in the media. Joint preparation and, hence, joint ownership of such guidelines between policy-makers, experts in the field and media personnel is essential.

Concluding comments

In concluding this book, we think it is essential to highlight what we consider to be key needs in this field. We will first highlight the needs related to improving clinical care of adolescents, including those who have self-harmed. We then turn to what we believe are important research needs that should be addressed. Finally, we underline the important responsibility that society has in relation to self-harm and suicidal behaviour in adolescents.

Clinical needs

There are some important aspects of clinical practice that need to be addressed in terms of improving the prevention and management of adolescent self-harm.

Attention needs to be paid to the problems that adolescents face and the management of such problems in the training of medical students, junior doctors, nurses and other healthcare professionals. In particular, these professionals need to be made fully aware of the difficulties that adolescents may have in accessing or otherwise dealing with clinical agencies. They also need training in the skills required to be able to interact effectively with adolescents.

General practice staff need to be particularly aware of the needs of adolescents, and attention should be paid to ensuring that practices are attractive to adolescents. Specific staff within a practice might take on particular responsibility for management of adolescents with psychosocial problems.

Hospital emergency department services need to be organised in an adolescent-friendly way, such that adolescents who present with deliberate self-harm or suicidal ideas can receive appropriate care.

Deliberate self-harm services in general hospitals, which should become the norm in all large hospitals, should include staff who have appropriate skills and take a special interest in adolescents who present following deliberate self-harm.

Prompt and detailed assessment should be conducted with all adolescents presenting to hospital following deliberate self-harm, including those who do not require admission to a hospital bed.

Further attention needs to be paid to the development and evaluation of effective treatments that might be utilised in the aftercare of adolescents who have presented with deliberate self-harm and in the management of adolescents at risk of self-harm or suicide. Such developments need to include attention to approaches that can help with difficulties of problem-solving that many such adolescents have, the needs of adolescents who engage in repeated self-harm, and those who have specific problems, such as family difficulties, substance misuse problems and behavioural disturbances. In view of the association between sexual abuse and the risk of repeated self-harm and the possible development of other coping difficulties, attention also needs to be paid to development and evaluation of treatments for abused adolescents. Intensive treatment, such as dialectical behaviour therapy, also requires evaluation in this population. Dialectical behaviour therapy has shown promising results in adults, and there are encouraging signs that it may be helpful for adolescents. Other approaches, including individual and family therapy, also require evaluation in such adolescents.

Research needs

Although much is now known about adolescents who present to hospital with deliberate self-harm, there is room for more investigation of those who engage in this behaviour in the community and do not come to clinical attention. In this book, we have focused a good deal on the results of our large-scale schools study, which had this very objective. However, other types of investigation of this kind are likely to be helpful. In particular, there is a need for longitudinal studies in which adolescents who are identified at the community level as having engaged in deliberate self-harm or being at risk of such behaviour are followed up in order to determine their outcome, in particular those who engage in further self-harm and suicidal behaviour and those who improve. The factors associated with such outcomes can then be identified. Deliberate self-harm by adolescents is clearly not an insignificant issue. A longitudinal study from New Zealand has shown that a substantial proportion of adolescents who engage in deliberate self-harm will engage in further such behaviour in young adulthood (Fergusson et al., 2005b).

Further work is required to investigate the mechanisms involved in the apparent contagious nature of self-harm, especially self-cutting, and to identify those adolescents who are most vulnerable to being influenced by exposure to self-harm by others.

We have highlighted the need for development of treatments for adolescents who have engaged in deliberate self-harm. The evaluation of treatments in this area is complex (Arensman et al., 2001). However, large-scale evaluative studies of new treatment approaches are required. These may need to be conducted as multi-centre studies in order to ensure inclusion of sufficient numbers of adolescents to fully test out the effectiveness of a particular approach.

We have indicated the extent to which schools should be an important focus for preventive efforts. Prevention programmes such as those that we have outlined require large-scale evaluation before being introduced more generally. In addition, where screening is being utilised to identify adolescents at risk, this also requires very careful evaluation, especially in view of the potential negative side effects for some adolescents.

Specific prevention initiatives aimed at adolescents should be investigated. An example of this is the evaluation of the legislation to restrict pack sizes of analgesics that was introduced in the UK in 1998. Careful evaluation has shown that this approach has been effective (Hawton et al., 2004b). Further initiatives require similar investigation.

The characteristics and needs of specific subgroups of adolescents involved in deliberate self-harm need to be studied. Examples include adolescents from ethnic minority groups, adolescents with sexual orientation concerns and adolescents who have been subjected to bullying.

Further work is required to investigate the role of the media in encouraging self-harming behaviour. This includes evaluation of the impact of specific media stimuli in which suicidal behaviour is portrayed or reported. In addition, we need more sophisticated evaluation of the ways in which media attention to suicidal behaviour can modify how adolescents react to problem situations. Finally, the potential role of the media in prevention of suicidal behaviour is an area of enormous potential importance that has so far received very little attention.

The role of the Internet in relation to both facilitation and prevention of suicidal behaviour is under-researched. We know very little about the ways in which adolescents make use of the Internet in help-seeking. We know even less about whether particular Internet sites or types of Internet presentation might encourage suicidal behaviour in adolescents.

Societal needs

One might regard the extent of self-harm and suicidal behaviour by young people in a society as reflecting the extent to which that society cares for and cherishes its young people. Levels of self-harm and suicidal behaviour are far higher in young people in many societies than they were three or four decades ago. There has been much debate about the reason for this. One obvious but important conclusion is that the problem of self-harm and suicidal behaviour among adolescents needs to be fully recognised within society. If there is adequate recognition of this problem, then this should lead to prioritisation of efforts to understand more about it, to develop preventive initiatives, to ensure that adequate clinical services for adolescents are available, attractive and staffed by knowledgeable individuals, to support helplines for adolescents in need, and to address issues and threats posed by the Internet and other aspects of the media.

It is largely with these needs in mind that we have written this book. We hope that it will make a significant contribution to the knowledge of readers about the problem of deliberate self-harm in adolescents and, hence, to achievement of at least some of the needs and goals that we have highlighted.

Guidelines Used in the Schools Study for Categorising Respondents' Descriptions of Deliberate Self-harm

Definition

The definition of deliberate self-harm (DSH) used was an act with a non-fatal outcome in which an individual deliberately:

(1)   initiates behaviour (such as self-cutting, hanging) that they intend to cause self-harm; and/or

(2)   ingests a substance in excess of the prescribed or generally recognised therapeutic dose; and/or

(3)   ingests a recreational/illicit drug[1] in an act that the person regarded as self-harm; and/or

(4)   ingests a non-ingestible substance or object.

This definition includes the following behaviour:

(1)   self-cutting (SC), hanging or strangulation (HA), suffocation (S), jumping or throwing self (J/T), electrocution (E), self-battery (SB), alcohol (AL), burning (B), inhalation/sniffing (I), starvation (SN), stopping of medication (SM), shooting (SH), drowning (D)

(2)   overdose (OD)

(3)   consuming a recreational drug (RD) (when the person actually regarded this as self-harm). The drug type consumed should be indicated: cocaine/crack (C), marijuana/cannabis (M), ecstasy (X), opiates/heroin (O), LSD/acid (L), amphetamine/speed (A), nature of the drug uncertain or unrecognisable (U)

---

1   For illicit/recreational drugs, ingestion of any amount was considered to be in excess of the prescribed or generally recognised therapeutic dose.

(4)   non-ingestible substance or object (NISO).

The guidelines on pages 194–200 were used for categorising respondents' answers to the question below:

When was the last time you took an overdose or tried to harm yourself?

☐ Less than a month ago

☐ Between a month and a year ago

☐ More than a year ago

Describe what you did to yourself on that occasion. Please give as much detail as you can – for example, the name of the drug taken in an overdose.

Use of the word 'tried' in the description

Where a respondent mentioned that he or she *tried* to do something, this was included under DSH. The reason for this is that the word 'tried' appeared in the wording of the question and, therefore, respondents may have picked up on the word in their response, e.g.

> I tried to slash my wrists with a Stanley knife blade.
> [coded as definitely DSH, SC]

Multiple methods mentioned

Multiple methods were all coded unless it was clear that the respondent was referring to more than one self-harm episode in their description. All methods in the following descriptions would have been coded:

> Took 30 ecstasy tablets and drank a litre of vodka with it.
> [coded as definitely DSH, OD, AL]

> Slit wrists and arms with razor, overdosed on paracetamol.
> [coded as definitely DSH, SC, OD]

> Cut self, suffocated self to a point.
> [coded as definitely DSH, SC, S]

If multiple methods were reported and they clearly occurred during different
self-harm episodes, then only the most recent method was coded, e.g.

> Slit my arm ages ago, was drunk. Overdosed in Strepsils three times, two
> weeks ago.
> [coded as definitely DSH, OD]

If it was impossible to determine which episode was the most recent, but it was clear
that the methods reported were employed during different self-harm episodes then
the first episode described was coded, e.g.

> I tried to slit my wrists on two occasions, I also tried to strangle myself with
> my school tie.
> [coded definitely DSH, SC]

> I took a packet of paracetamol and took over half the packet. I have tried to
> jump from high places and I tried a knife to my stomach.
> [coded as definitely DSH, OD]

Alcohol

For alcohol to be coded as a method of deliberate self-harm, it must have been indicated clearly by the respondent as being used for the purposes of self-harm. It was
not enough for respondents to simply mention that they had been drinking at the
time of the self-harm episode, e.g.

> I do not know what drug I took, but I was under a lot of pressure. I was
> drinking alcohol at the time. I took an overdose of pills and decided to drink
> because of pressure and stress.
> [coded as definitely DSH, OD]

> I overdosed on paracetamol and took a whole bottle of pills, but I was pissed.
> [coded as definitely DSH, OD]

I had been drinking a lot and I went into the bathroom and took a lot of pills
– I do not know how many or what they were.
[coded as definitely DSH, OD]

I had a bit of alcohol and cut myself on my arm using a kitchen knife.
[coded as definitely DSH, SC]

None of the above descriptions would have been coded for alcohol being used as a method of DSH. Although the respondents mentioned that they had been drinking at the time of the DSH episode, they did not describe/or imply alcohol as a DSH method.

Episodes that would have been coded as including alcohol as a method of DSH include the following:

Took an alcohol and drug overdose, vodka and unknown (believed to be morphine) taken from a friend.
[coded as definitely DSH AL, RD(O)]

I took paracetamol with alcohol.
[coded as definitely DSH, AL, OD]

I drank loads of Skol and Diamond White.
[coded as definitely DSH, AL]

Recreational drugs

In response to the question 'Describe what you did to yourself', ingestion of any amount of an illicit/recreational drug was considered to be an overdose of the named illicit/recreational drug. Recreational drugs mentioned in the description were classified as 'RD'. The type of recreational drug used was coded, e.g. 'I took crack' was coded as RD(C).

In some cases, it was not clear what the substance mentioned was. These cases were coded as RD (U), e.g. 'Sleepy drug available from the M.Corp' was coded as RD(U). However, if the respondent mentioned that they were on something while they engaged in DSH, then the illicit substance was not coded, e.g.

I was on cannabis and took too much paracetamol.
[coded as definitely DSH, OD]

After taking hash, I raided the medicine cabinet.
[coded as definitely DSH, OD]

Starvation

For deliberate starvation to be included as a method of DSH, the respondent had to indicate that it was used for the purpose of self-harm, e.g.

> I have not taken a drug overdose, but I have starved myself to the point of not being able to concentrate in school or work to a normal level.
> [coded as definitely DSH, SN].

Eating disorders such as bulimia nervosa and other specific eating disorder symptoms are not included, e.g.

> I'm not sure if this counts, but I have made myself sick. After a meal I excuse myself and stick my fingers down my throat.

> I made myself throw up because I felt fat.

Stopping of medication

Cessation of medication when this is likely to cause harm was included, e.g.

> I stopped my insulin.
> [coded as definitely DSH, SM]

> I refused to use my inhaler.
> [coded as definitely DSH, SM]

No deliberate self-help information given

Sometimes, respondents answered this question with an explanation of the reason behind their actions. Alternatively, some respondents did not actually explain what it was that they did. On both occasions, the description was be classified as 'No DSH information given', e.g.

> I didn't try to overdose.

> I didn't overdose, I just hurt myself.

Both of these individuals were saying that they did not take an overdose. It is, however, possible that the respondents could have engaged in some other means of deliberate self-harm. These descriptions were, therefore, classified as 'no DSH information given'.

Other respondents did not wish or were unable to give details of the self-harm episode, e.g.

> Can't remember.

This respondent was saying that he or she did not want or was unable to tell us about his or her last episode, so the description was classified as 'no DSH information given'.

Some respondents supplied a reason for their behaviour but did not give details of the actual episode, e.g.

> I got involved with the wrong people and after being persuaded, I got to like the idea and so did it a few times.

This respondent provided us with a reason for his or her behaviour but did not explain what it was he or she did. This was, therefore, coded as 'no DSH information given'.

Finally, some respondents indicated that they had engaged in self-harm behaviour by answering 'Yes' to the question 'Have you ever deliberately taken an overdose (e.g. of pills or other medication) or tried to harm yourself in some other way (such as cut yourself?).' However, they failed to give any details of their last episode. Therefore, these descriptions were coded as 'no DSH information given'.

Third party intervention

Sometimes, respondents mentioned that a third party disturbed them. In these cases, the descriptions were classified as definitely self-harm, e.g.

> I tried to take an overdose of paracetamol, but my sister found me before I took too many so there was no serious harm.
> [coded as definitely DSH, OD]

> Ran out in front of a lorry on the A road outside my house, but best friend ran out after me and pushed me to the side.
> [coded as definitely DSH, J/T]

> I tried to hang myself with a dressing gown rope, but a parent caught me.
> [coded as definitely DSH, HA]

Not deliberate self-harm

Sometimes, respondents answered the question about self-harm inappropriately. If the description offered did not conform to our definition (see the first two pages of this appendix), then it was coded as not DSH. For example, in the following case, the respondent appeared to have misunderstood the question and answered it with an explanation of what she did whenever she hurt herself:

> Paracetamol for headache. Pain killers – if I had a sore throat or gum pain. TCP when I cut myself, for example, cut my finger with the knife by accident when I was cutting something.

In the cases below, the respondents said that they threatened to cut themselves, but the implication was that they did not go through with it. The descriptions were therefore coded as not DSH.

> I threatened to cut myself with a knife.

> Tried to slit my wrists, I put a knife to my wrist and went to cut them, but realised it was stupid and stopped.

If the description offered by the respondents was clearly not DSH, or it appeared that the respondent had been taking therapeutic doses of medication, then the description was coded as not DSH.

> I was very upset, so I had a aspirin.

> I had a headache and took two tablets a month for it.

> I bit my nails off along with the surrounding skins, causing them to bleed.

Information Sheet Given to Participants After Completing the Questionnaire

Useful contacts

If you have any problems, mental or physical, that are really worrying you, **see your doctor (GP) as soon as possible**. They're there to help with your problems.

If you can't or don't want to talk to your family, friends or teachers about problems or worries, you could call a helpline. Helplines can provide expert advice, information or a friendly ear. Phone numbers for some helplines are listed below, along with web sites and e-mail addresses (if they have one):

Alateen: for young people with alcoholic parents and carers.
020 7403 0888 – 24 hours a day, 7 days a week
www.hexnet.co.uk/alanon/alateen

Anti-Bullying Campaign: confidential help and advice if you are being bullied or are a bully.
020 7378 1446 – 10am to 4pm, Monday to Friday

Brook Advisory Centres: free confidential advice and counselling on emotional and sexual problems, contraception and pregnancy.
0800 0185 023 – 9am to 5pm, Monday to Friday
www.brook.org.uk

ChildLine: free confidential helpline for young people in trouble or danger.
0800 1111 – 24 hours a day, 7 days a week
www.childline.org.uk

Eating Disorders Youth Helpline: help, support and information for those whose lives are affected by eating disorders.
0845 634 7650 – 4pm to 6pm, Monday to Friday
www.edauk.com

London Lesbian and Gay Switchboard: for anyone who needs support, help or information on love, life, safer sex and practically anything else.
020 7837 7324 – 24 hours a day, 7 days a week
www.llgs.org.uk

Mind Info Line: information on all aspects of mental distress.
0845 766 0163 – 9.15am to 4.45pm, Monday to Friday
www.mind.org.uk
email: info@mind.org.uk

National Drugs Helpline: information, advice and counselling on any drug worries, whether about yourself or anyone else.
0800 77 66 00 – 24 hours a day, 7 days a week
www.talktofrank.com

Samaritans: offers free emotional support to anyone going through a crisis.
08457 90 90 90 – 24 hours a day, 7 days a week
www.samaritans.org.uk
email: jo@samaritans.org

YoungMinds: information and advice for anyone concerned about mental health matters.
020 7336 8445
www.youngminds.org.uk

APPENDIX III

Self-harm: Guidelines for School Staff

These guidelines (pp.202–223, marked ✓) may be photocopied for use by teachers and professionals supporting young people, but any material copied or used must be acknowledged and fully referenced.

These guidelines were produced as the result of collaboration between Oxfordshire Education Department, Oxford Samaritans, Oxfordshire Mental Healthcare Trust and the Department of Social and Health Care. They were written by the Adolescent Self-Harm Steering Group to help school staff to support young people who harm themselves.

The guidelines are primarily intended for use in secondary schools and should be read in conjunction with the Area Child Protection Committee (ACPC) guidelines 2002. Anyone wishing to publish excerpts from the guidelines should contact:

>**Oxfordshire Adolescent Self-Harm Forum**
>c/o Highfield Family and Adolescent Unit
>The Warneford Hospital
>Warneford Lane
>Headington
>Oxford OX3 75X

Contents

What is self-harm and how common is it?

Self-harm is any behaviour such as self-cutting, swallowing objects, taking an overdose, hanging or running in front of a car where the intent is to deliberately cause self-harm.

Some people who self-harm have a strong desire to kill themselves. However, there are other factors that motivate people to self-harm, including a desire to escape an unbearable situation or intolerable emotional pain, to reduce tension, to express hostility, to induce guilt or to increase caring from others. Even if the intent to die is not high, self-harming behaviour may express a powerful sense of despair and needs to be taken seriously. Moreover, some people who do not intend to kill themselves may do so because they do not realise the seriousness of the method they have chosen or because they do not get help in time.

Over the past 40 years, there has been a large increase in the number of young people who deliberately harm themselves. A large community study in the UK found that among 15- to 16-year-olds, approximately 6.9 per cent (3.2% males, 11.2% females) had self-harmed in the past year (Hawton *et al.*, 2002).

What causes self-harm?

The following risk factors, particularly in combination, may make a young person vulnerable to self-harm:

Individual factors:

- depression/anxiety
- poor communication skills
- low self-esteem
- poor problem-solving skills
- hopelessness
- impulsivity
- drug or alcohol abuse.

Family factors:

- unreasonable expectations
- neglect or abuse (physical, sexual or emotional)
- poor parental relationships and arguments
- depression, deliberate self-harm or suicide in the family.

Social factors:

- difficulty in making relationships/loneliness
- persistent bullying or peer rejection
- easy availability of drugs, medication or other methods of self-harm.

A number of factors may trigger the self-harm incident, including:

- family relationship difficulties (the most common trigger for younger adolescents)
- difficulties with peer relationships, e.g. break-up of relationship (the most common trigger for older adolescents)
- bullying
- significant trauma, e.g. bereavement, abuse
- self-harm behaviour in other students (contagion effect)
- self-harm portrayed or reported in the media
- difficult times of the year, e.g. anniversaries
- trouble in school or with the police
- feeling under pressure from families, school or peers to conform/achieve
- exam pressure
- times of change, e.g. parental separation/divorce.

Warning signs

There may be a change in behaviour of the young person that is associated with self-harm or other serious emotional difficulties, such as:

- changes in eating/sleeping habits
- increased isolation from friends/family
- changes in activity and mood, e.g. more aggressive than usual
- lowering of academic grades
- talking about self-harming or suicide
- abusing drugs or alcohol

- becoming socially withdrawn
- expressing feelings of failure, uselessness or loss of hope
- giving away possessions.

Examples of self-harming behaviour

- cutting
- taking an overdose of tablets
- swallowing hazardous materials or substances
- burning, either physically or chemically
- over/undermedicating, e.g. misuse of insulin
- punching/hitting/bruising
- hair-pulling/skin-picking/head-banging
- episodes of alcohol/drug abuse or over/undereating at times may be acts of deliberate self-harm.

Self-harm can be a transient behaviour in young people that is triggered by particular stresses and resolves fairly quickly, or it may be part of a longer-term pattern of behaviour that is associated with more serious emotional/psychiatric difficulties. Where a number of underlying risk factors are present, the risk of further self-harm is greater.

Some young people get caught up in mild repetitive self-harm, such as scratching, which is often done in a peer group. In this case, it may be helpful to take a low-key approach, avoiding escalation, although at the same time being vigilant for signs of more serious self-harm.

What keeps self-harm going?

Once self-harm, particularly cutting, is established, it may be difficult to stop. Self-harm can have a number of functions for the student and it becomes a way of coping, for example:

- reduction in tension (safety valve)
- distraction from problems
- form of escape
- outlet for anger and rage
- opportunity to feel
- way of punishing self
- way of taking control

- care-eliciting behaviour
- means of getting identity with a peer group
- non-verbal communication (e.g. of abusive situation)
- suicidal act.

Cycle of self-harm/cutting

When a person inflicts pain upon him- or herself, the body responds by producing endorphins, a natural pain-reliever that gives temporary relief or a feeling of peace. The addictive nature of this feeling can make the stopping of self-harm difficult. Young people who self-harm still feel pain, but some say the physical pain is easier to stand than the emotional/mental pain that led to the self-harm initially (Figure AIII.1).

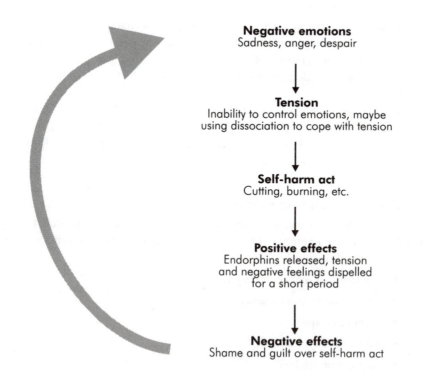

Negative emotions
Sadness, anger, despair

↓

Tension
Inability to control emotions, maybe using dissociation to cope with tension

↓

Self-harm act
Cutting, burning, etc.

↓

Positive effects
Endorphins released, tension and negative feelings dispelled for a short period

↓

Negative effects
Shame and guilt over self-harm act

AIII.1 Cycle of self-harm

Coping strategies

Replacing the cutting or other self-harm with other safer activities can be a positive way of coping with the tension. What works depends on the reasons behind the self-harm. Activities that involve the emotions intensively can be helpful. Examples of ways of coping include:

- writing, drawing and talking about feelings
- writing a letter expressing feelings, which need not be sent
- contacting a friend or family member
- ringing a helpline
- going into a field and screaming
- hitting a pillow or soft object
- listening to loud music
- going for a walk/run or other forms of physical exercise
- getting out of the house and going to a public place, e.g. a cinema
- reading a book
- keeping a diary
- using stress-management techniques, such as relaxation
- having a bath
- looking after an animal.

In the longer term, the young person may need to develop ways of understanding and dealing with the underlying emotions and beliefs. Regular counselling/ therapy may be helpful. Family support is likely to be an important part of this.

It may also help if the young person joins a group activity such as a youth club, a keep-fit class or a school-based club that will provide opportunities for the person to develop friendships and feel better about him- or herself. Learning stress-management techniques, ways to keep safe and how to relax may also be useful.

Reactions of school staff

School staff members may experience a range of feelings in response to self-harm in a young person, such as anger, sadness, shock, disbelief, guilt, helplessness, disgust and rejection. It is important for all work colleagues to have an opportunity to discuss the impact that self-harm has on them personally. The type and nature of the forums where these issues are discussed will vary between schools.

Students may present with injuries to first-aid or reception staff. It is important that these frontline staff are aware that an injury may be self-inflicted and that they pass on any concerns.

The urge to escape difficulties

For some young people, self-harm expresses the strong desire to escape from a conflict or unhappiness at home and to live elsewhere. Injuring oneself can achieve a temporary respite if it entails a hospital admission or a short break at the home of a friend or relative. The young person may request admission to foster care or a residential home, and parents may doubt their ability to cope at this stage. Entering care carries with it many long-term disadvantages and increased vulnerability for the young person. It is far preferable to try to support the young person and family members in finding a resolution to their difficulties than to separate them further. However, if you believe that a young person would be at serious risk of abuse in returning home, then you should consult a social worker for advice.

How to help

First-line help

- When you recognise signs of distress, try to find ways of talking with the young person about how he or she is feeling.

- Build up a full picture of the young person's life by talking to his or her form tutor, year head and any other adults who come into contact with him or her. Find out the person's particular strengths and vulnerabilities.

- What appears to be important for many young people is having someone to talk to who *listens properly* and does not judge. This person may be, for example, a mentor, counsellor, youth worker, school health nurse, teacher, personal Connexions adviser, special educational needs coordinator, behaviour support teacher, educational social worker or educational psychologist.

- It is important that all attempts of suicide or deliberate self-harm are taken seriously. All mention of suicidal thoughts should be noticed and the young person listened to carefully.

- If you find a young person who has self-harmed, e.g. by overdosing or self-cutting, try to keep calm, give reassurance and follow the first-aid guidelines as directed by school policy. In the case of an overdose of tablets, however small, advice must be obtained from a medical practitioner (GP or accident and emergency department).

- Take a non-judgemental attitude towards the young person. Try to reassure the person that you understand that the self-harm is helping him or her to cope at the moment and you want to help. Explain that you need to tell someone. Try to work out together who is the best person to tell (see Confidentiality on p.210).

- Discuss with the young person the importance of letting his or her parents know and any fears he or she may have about this.

- Contact the person's parents, unless there are particular reasons why they should not be contacted, and discuss the school's concern. Give the parents the parents' fact sheet (see p.220) and help the parents to understand the self-harm so that they can be supportive to the young person.

- Suggest to the parents a referral to the GP. Ask for feedback from the parents so that the school can work with the young person.

- The Social and Health Care Department (previously social services) should be informed if the young person discloses child protection concerns. Follow the Area Child Protection Committee Guidelines, 2002. Document any conversations you have had with the social worker. Record who you spoke to, the time, date and any advice they have given you to follow.

- If your contact with the young person reveals that his or her future health and development are at serious risk, then consult the Social and Health Care Department.

- To make a social work referral to the Social and Health Care Department, use the form developed by social services to document your knowledge/observations of the young person and his or her family and send it to the young person's local Child and Families Assessment team. Copies of this form should be available from the school or the Social and Health Care Department. You should inform the young person and his or her parents if you are making a social work referral, unless it would compromise someone's safety to do so.

- If other agencies are already involved with the young person, then it may be important to liaise with these agencies and work together.

- Follow up the parents' meeting with a letter indicating your concern (an example is provided on p.216).

- Have crisis telephone numbers available and easily accessible to young people.

- Follow the school policy of informing the senior management/leadership team of your concerns.

- Record any incident (an example is provided on p.217).

- Seek support for yourself if necessary.

Longer-term support of a young person who self-harms

It may be appropriate to provide more ongoing support within school for a young person who is self-harming. It is important that those who undertake this role feel able to do so and are supported fully by management.

Understanding the self-harm

It may be helpful to explore with the young person what led to the self-harm – the feelings, thoughts and behaviour involved. This can help the young person make sense of the self-harm and develop alternative ways of coping.

Confidentiality

Confidentiality is a key concern for young people, and they need to know that it may not be possible for their support member of staff to offer complete confidentiality. If you consider that a young person is at serious risk of harming him- or herself or others, then confidentiality cannot be kept. It is important not to make promises of confidentiality that you cannot keep, even though the young person may put pressure on you to do so. If this is explained at the outset of any meeting, then the young person can make an informed decision as to how much information he or she wishes to divulge.

Strategies to help

- Arrange a mutually convenient time and place to meet.
- At the start of the meeting, set a time limit.
- Make sure the young person understands the limits of your confidentiality.
- Encourage the young person to talk about what has led him or her to self-harm.
- Remember that listening is a vital part of this process.
- Support the young person in beginning to take the steps necessary to keep him or her safe and to reduce the self-injury (if he or she wishes to), e.g.
  - washing implements used to cut
  - avoiding alcohol if it is likely to lead to self-injury
  - taking better care of injuries (the school health nurse may be helpful here).
- Help the young person to learn how to express his or her feelings in other ways, e.g. talking, writing, drawing or using safer alternatives (as described earlier).
- Help the young person to build up self-esteem.
- Help the young person to find his or her own way of managing problems, e.g.
  - if the person dislikes him- or herself, begin working on what he or she does like.

- ° if life at home is impossible, begin working on how to talk to parents/carers.
- Help the young person to identify his or her own support network (see p.218).
- Offer information about support agencies. Remember that some Internet sites may contain inappropriate information.

Further considerations

- Record any meetings with the young person. Include an agreed action plan, including dates, times and any concerns you have. Document who else has been informed of any information.

- It is important to encourage young people to let you know if one of their group is in trouble, upset or shows signs of harming. Friends can worry about betraying confidences, so they need to know that self-harm can be dangerous to life and that by seeking help and advice for a friend they are taking a responsible action.

- The peer group of a young person who self-harms may value the opportunity to talk to an adult, either individually or in a small group.

Response of supportive members of staff

For those who are supporting young people who self-harm, it is important to be clear with each individual how often and for how long you are going to see them, i.e. the boundaries need to be clear. It can be easy to get caught up in providing too much help, because of one's own anxiety. However, the young person needs to learn to take responsibility for his or her self-harm.

If you find that the self-harm upsets you, it may be helpful to be honest with the young person. However, be clear that you can deal with your own feelings and try to avoid the young person feeling blamed. The young person probably already feels low in mood and has a poor self-image; your anger or upset may add to his or her negative feelings. However, your feelings matter too. You will need the support of your colleagues and management if you are to listen effectively to young people's difficulties.

Issues regarding contagion

When a young person is self-harming, it is important to be vigilant in case close contacts of the individual are also self-harming. Occasionally, schools discover that a number of students in the same peer group are harming themselves. Self-harm can become an acceptable way of dealing with stress within a peer group and may increase peer identity. This can cause considerable anxiety, both in school staff and in other young people.

Each individual may have different reasons for self-harming and should be given the opportunity for one-to-one support. However, it may also be helpful to discuss the matter openly with the group of young people involved. In general, it is not advisable to offer regular group support for young people who self-harm.

Support/training aspects for staff

Staff members giving support to young people who self-harm may experience all sorts of reactions to this behaviour in young people, such as anger, helplessness and rejection. It is helpful for staff to have an opportunity to talk this through with work colleagues or senior management.

Staff members with this role should take the opportunity to attend training days on self-harm or read relevant literature. Liaison with the local specialist child and adolescent mental health service may be helpful.

General aspects of prevention of self-harm

An important part of prevention of self-harm is having a supportive environment in the school that is focused on building self-esteem and encouraging healthy peer relationships. An effective anti-bullying policy and a means of identifying and supporting young people with emotional difficulties is an important aspect of this. The checklist of procedures and practices on pp.214–215 can help in the management and prevention of self-harm.

Helping young people who self-harm

Young person is self-harming

↓

Member of staff informed/discovers a student with problem
Member of staff to talk to young person
In an emergency, school staff to follow first-aid guidelines

↓

Each member of staff to follow the school policy regarding informing the senior management/leadership team (this allows the staff member to gain support of colleagues), e.g. head of year, child protection designated teacher, head teacher, etc.
Consideration given to informing parents

↓

Discussion with relevant professionals involved with young person, e.g. Connexions, school health nurse, educational psychologist, educational social worker

↓

Consultation with Social and Health Care or Specialist Child
and Adolescent Mental Health Service may be helpful

↓

Meeting with parents to inform and discuss concerns:
- follow up the meeting with a letter (see p.216)
- give crisis/helpline details to parents and young person
- give fact sheet to parents and carers (see p.219–220)
- refer to Child Protection Guidelines and act accordingly (note confidentiality guidelines)

↓

GP sees young person to assess appropriate help required
(Ideally, feedback given to school)

↓   ↓

Continue work at primary-care level with supervision/support	Send referral to Specialist child/adolescent mental health service or other services such as family therapy or counselling for children who have been sexually abused
↓	↓
Regularly review and evaluate progress/concerns with young person Consider range of interventions, e.g. develop peer support network, family support, education interventions, school counselling	Referral to more intensive service as required

↓

Referral to Specialist Child/Adolescent Mental Health Service if GP feels it is required

Optimal conditions: link established between young person, parent, school and ongoing support

Checklist for schools: supporting the development of effective practice

School policy

The school has a policy or protocol for supporting students who are, or are ☐ at risk, of self-harming. The school governors have approved this.

The Oxfordshire Self-harm Guidelines have been approved by the school ☐ governors.

Training

All new members of staff receive an induction on child-protection proce- ☐ dures and setting boundaries around confidentiality.

All members of staff receive regular training on child-protection proce- ☐ dures.

The following staff groups – reception staff, first-aid staff, technicians, ☐ dinner supervisors – receive sufficient training and preparation for their roles.

Staff members with pastoral roles (heads of year, child protection ☐ co-ordinator, etc.) have access to training in identifying and supporting students who self-harm.

Communication

The school has clear open channels of communication that allow informa- ☐ tion to be passed up, down and across the system.

All members of staff know to whom they can go if they discover a young ☐ person who is self-harming.

The senior management team is fully aware of the contact that reception, ☐ first-aid staff, technicians and dinner supervisors have with young people and the types of issue they may come across.

Time is made available to listen to and support the concerns of staff ☐ members on a regular basis.

Support for staff/students

Staff members know the different agency members who visit the school, □
e.g. school counsellors, Connexions personal advisers, etc.

Male members of staff are supported in considering their responses to girls □
whom they notice are self-harming.

Staff members know how to access support for themselves and students. □

Students know to whom they can go for help. □

School ethos

The school has a culture that encourages young people to talk and adults to □
listen and believe.

Sample of letter to parents

Dear [parent/carer]

Thank you for coming to school to discuss ....

....

....

After our recent meeting, I am writing to express concern about ....'s safety and welfare. The recent incident of self-harm (or threat to self-harm) by .... suggests that he/she may need professional help.

I recommend that you visit your local GP for advice and help.

We will continue to provide support within the school community but would appreciate any information that you feel would help us to do this as effectively as possible.

If there is anything else we can do to help .... please contact me.

Yours sincerely,

[Name]
[Title]

Sample of an incident form to be used when a young person self-harms

School/college   Date of report
Staff member   Position

Young person's name
Age   Gender   Year   Special needs

Incident...
....
....
....

Date and time of occurence ....

Action taken by school personnel...
....
....

Decision made with respect to contacting parents and reasons for decision
....
....
....

Recommendations..
....
....

Follow-up ....
....
....

My safety net

There are different types of people in our lives. Try to identify some people in each of the groups below that you would feel comfortable talking to:

- family and close friends
- friends and people you see every day
- helplines and professional people you could go to for help.

Also, write into the space below the safety net the things that you can do yourself to cope with difficult feelings and keep yourself safe.

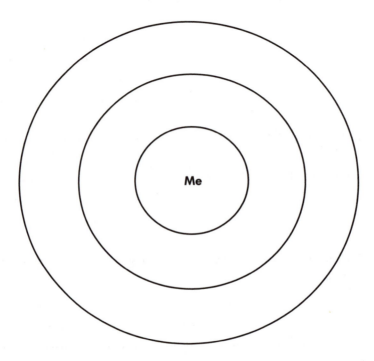

Things I can do myself to cope with difficult feelings

Fact sheet on self-harm for parents/carers

It can be difficult to find out that someone you care about is harming him- or herself. As a parent/carer, you may feel angry, shocked, guilty and upset. These reactions are normal, but what the person you care about really needs is support from you. The person needs you to stay calm and to listen to him or her. The reason someone self-harms is to help him or her cope with very difficult feelings that build up and cannot be expressed. The person needs to find a less harmful way of coping.

What is self-harm?

Self-harm is any behaviour such as self-cutting, swallowing objects, taking an overdose, hanging or running in front of a car where the intent is to deliberately cause harm to self.

How common is self-harm?

Over the past 40 years, there has been a large increase in the number of young people who harm themselves. A large community study found that among 15- to 16-year-olds, approximately 7 per cent had self-harmed in the previous year.

Is it just attention-seeking?

Some people who self-harm have a desire to kill themselves. However, there are many other factors that lead people to self-harm, including a desire to escape, to reduce tension, to express hostility, to make someone feel guilty or to increase caring from others. Even if the young person does not intend to commit suicide, self-harming behaviour may express a strong sense of despair and needs to be taken seriously. It is not just attention-seeking behaviour.

Why do young people harm themselves?

All sorts of upsetting events can trigger self-harm, such as arguments with family, break-up of a relationship, failure in exams and bullying at school. Sometimes, several stresses occur over a short period of time and one more incident is the final straw.

Young people who have emotional or behavioural problems or low self-esteem can be particularly at risk from self-harm. Suffering a bereavement or serious rejection can also increase the risk. Sometimes, young people try to escape their problems by taking drugs or alcohol. This only makes the situation worse. For some people, self-harm is a desperate attempt to show others that something is wrong in their lives.

What can you do to help?

- Keep an open mind.
- Make the time to listen.
- Help the person find different ways of coping.
- Go with the person to get the right kind of help as quickly as possible.

Some people you can contact for help, advice and support are:

- your family doctor
- Young Minds Parents Information Service: tel. 0800 018 2138
- Samaritans: tel. 08457 90 90 90
- PAPYRUS HOPELine UK tel. 0870 170 4000
- MIND Info Line: tel. 0845 766 0163 (self-help books also available)
- Youth Access: tel. 020 8772 9900
- school health nurse
- health visitor.

Information sheet on self-harm for young people

What is self-harm?

Self-harm is where someone does something to deliberately hurt him- or herself. This may include cutting parts of the body, burning, hitting or taking an overdose.

How many young people self-harm?

A large study in the UK found that about 7 per cent (i.e. 7 out of every 100 people) of 15- to 16-year-olds had self-harmed in the past year.

Why do young people self-harm?

Self-harm is often a way of trying to cope with painful and confusing feelings. Difficult things that people who self-harm talk about include:

- feeling sad or feeling worried
- not feeling very good or confident about themselves
- being hurt by others: physically, sexually or emotionally
- feeling under a lot of pressure at school or at home
- losing someone close, such as someone dying or leaving.

When difficult or stressful things happen in a person's life, it can trigger self-harm. Upsetting events that might lead to self-harm include:

- arguments with family or friends
- break-up of a relationship
- failing, or thinking you are going to fail, exams
- being bullied.

Often, these things build up until the young person feels he or she cannot cope anymore. Self-harm can be a way of trying to deal with or escaping from these difficult feelings. It can also be a way of the person showing other people that something is wrong in his or her life.

How can you cope with self-harm?

Replacing the self-harm with other, safer, coping strategies can be a positive and more helpful way of dealing with difficult things in your life. Helpful strategies can include:

- finding someone to talk to about your feelings, such as a friend or family member
- talking to someone on the phone, e.g. you might want to ring a helpline

- writing and drawing about your feelings, because sometimes it can be hard to talk about feelings
- scribbling on and/or ripping up paper
- listening to music
- going for a walk, run or other kind of exercise
- getting out of the house and going somewhere where there are other people
- keeping a diary
- having a bath/using relaxing oils, e.g. lavender
- hitting a pillow or other soft object
- watching a favourite film.

Getting help

In the longer term, it is important that the young person learns to understand and deal with the causes of the stress that he or she feels. The support of someone who understands and will listen to you can be very helpful in facing difficult feelings:

- *At home:* parents, brother/sister or another trusted family member.
- *In school:* school counsellor, school nurse, teacher, teaching assistant or other member of staff.
- *GP:* you can talk to your GP about your difficulties and he or she can make a referral for counselling.
- *Help lines:*
    - Young Minds: tel. 020 7336 8445 or email enquiries@youngminds.org.uk
    - Samaritans: tel. 08457 90 90 90 or email jo@samaritans.org.uk
    - MIND Info Line: tel. 0845 766 0163 (self-help books are also available)
    - Youth Access: tel. 020 8772 9900.
- Information leaflet available through: www.nch.org.uk/self-harm.
- Another useful address is:

National Self Harm Network
PO Box 7264
Nottingham NG1 6WJ
www.nshn.co.uk

My friend has a problem: how can I help?

- You can really help by just being there, listening and giving support.

- Be open and honest. If you are worried about your friend's safety, you should tell an adult. Let your friend know that you are going to do this and you are doing it because you care about him or her.

- Encourage your friend to get help. You can go with your friend or tell someone he or she wants to know about it.

- Get information from telephone helplines, websites, a library, etc. This can help you understand what your friend is experiencing.

- Your friendship may be changed by the problem. You may feel bad that you can't help your friend enough or guilty if you have had to tell other people. These feelings are common and don't mean that you have done something wrong or not done enough.

- Your friend may get angry with you or tell you that you don't understand. It is important to try not to take this personally. Often, when people are feeling bad about themselves, they get angry with the people they are closest to.

- It can be difficult to look after someone who is having difficulties. It is important for you to to talk to an adult who can support you. You may not always be able to be there for your friend, and that's OK.

Acknowledgements

The Oxfordshire Adolescent Self-Harm Forum wishes to thank Chris Sey, Principal Education Psychologist, for facilitating the funding that allowed these guidelines to be produced and for all his ongoing support.

We are grateful to the following people for providing advice on the guidelines: Judith Atkinson, David Bingley, Simon Cornwell, Caroline Crosbie, Hannah Farncombe, Fran Fonseca, Vic Gore, Sue Harris, Keith Hawton, Francis Josephs, Chris Sey, Anna Turner and Tina Pegg.

The Oxfordshire Adolescent Self-Harm Steering Group comprises:

- Carrie Jackson, School Health Nurse. Project Coordinator
- Anne Stewart, Consultant Psychiatrist, Highfield
- Elisabeth Salisbury, Samaritans
- Karen Rodham, Centre for Suicide Research
- Tara Midgen, Educational Psychologist
- Tessa Cullen, Deputy Head of Student Services, Banbury School
- Claire Holdaway, Clinical Psychologist, Abingdon
- Linda Whitehead, Barnes Unit
- Sharon Codd, Counsellor, Barnes Unit.

Robson's Self Concept Scale (Short Version)

		Completely disagree	Disagree	Agree	Completely agree
1.	I'm glad I'm who I am	☐	☐	☐	☐
2.	There are lots of things I'd change about myself if I could	☐	☐	☐	☐
3.	It's pretty tough to be me	☐	☐	☐	☐
4.	I have a pleasant personality	☐	☐	☐	☐
5.	I have control over my own life	☐	☐	☐	☐
6.	Everyone seems much more confident and contented than me	☐	☐	☐	☐
7.	Even when I enjoy myself there doesn't seem much purpose to it all	☐	☐	☐	☐
8.	I can like myself even when others don't	☐	☐	☐	☐

Developed with the assistance of Dr Philip Robson from the original version of the Self Concept Scale (Robson, P. (1989) Development of a new self-report questionnaire to measure self-esteem. *Psychological Medicine 19*, 513–518).

Useful Contact Addresses in the UK for Young People with Problems, or their Friends or Relatives in Need of Advice

Alateen

Provides help for young people aged between 12 and 20 years who have relatives or friends with alcohol problems.

61 Great Dover Street
London SE1 4YF
Tel: 020 7403 0888
www.hexnet.co.uk/alanon/alateen.org

Anti-Bullying Campaign

Offers support, advice, information and understanding to parents whose children are being bullied at school and to children who are bullied.

185 Tower Bridge Road
London SE1 2UF
Tel: 020 7378 1446 (Mon–Fri, 10am–4pm)

Bristol Crisis Service for Women

National voluntary organisation that supports women in emotional distress, especially women who harm themselves.

PO Box 654
Bristol BS99 lXH
Tel: 0117 925 1119
www.users.zetnet.co.uk/BCSW/
Email: bcsw@btconnect.com

Brook Advisory Centres
Provides advice on pregnancy and contraception for young people up to the age of 25 years.

421 Highgate Studios
57–79 Highgate Road
London NW5 1TL
Tel: 0800 0185 023
www.brook.org.uk
Email: admin@brookecentres.org.uk

CALM (Campaign Against Living Miserably)
Confidential helpline service offering support and advice to young men under the age of 25 years who are at the start of depression.

Room 621, Gateway House
Piccadilly South
Manchester M60 7PL
Tel: 800 58 58 58 (seven days a week 5pm–3am)
www.comcarenet.co.uk/trafford/therapy/calm.htm
Email: info@comcarenet.co.uk

Child Bereavement Trust
Offers support to grieving family members of all ages.

Aston House
West Wycombe
High Wycombe
Bucks HP14 3AG
Tel: 0845 357 1000
www.childbereavement.org.uk
Email: enquiries@childbereavement.org.uk

ChildLine
Telephone helpline for children and adolescents.

Freepost 1111
London N1 0BR
Tel: 0800 1111
www.childline.org.uk

Cruse Bereavement Care

Promotes the well-being of bereaved people and aims to help those who are bereaved to understand their grief and cope with their loss.

Cruse House
126 Sheen Road
Richmond
Surrey TW9 1UR
Tel: 0870 167 1677
www.crusebereavementcare.org.uk
Email: helpline@crusebereavementcare.org.uk

Eating Disorders Association

Provides information on all aspects of eating disorders, including anorexia nervosa, bulimia nervosa, binge-eating disorder and related eating disorders.

First Floor, Wensum House
103 Prince of Wales Road
Norwich NR1 1DW
Adult helpline: 0845 634 1414
Youthline: 0845 634 7650
www.edauk.com
Email (adults): helpmail@edauk.com
Email (youthline): talkback@edauk.com

London Lesbian and Gay Switchboard

Provides an information, support and referral service for lesbians, gay men and bisexual people from all backgrounds.

PO Box 7324
London N1 9QS
Tel: 0207 837 7324
www.llgs.org.uk
Email: admin@llgs.org.uk

Mental Health Foundation

Aims to help people survive and recover from mental health problems and to prevent such problems.

London Office
9th Floor, Sea Containers House
20 Upper Ground
London SE1 9QB
Tel: 020 7803 1100
www.mentalheath.org.uk
Email: mhf@mhf.org.uk

National Self-Harm Network
Provides information and campaigns for people who self-harm.

PO BOX 7264
Nottingham NG1 6WJ
www.nshn.co.uk
Email: info@nshn.co.uk

Papyrus (Parents Association for the Prevention of Young Suicide)
Charity committed to suicide prevention, focusing on the emotional well-being of children, teenagers and young adults. Have a telephone helpline offering professional advice for anyone worried about a young person who may be suicidal.

Rossendale Hospital
Union Road
Rawtenstall
Lancashire BB4 6NE
Tel: 01706 214449
www.papyrus-uk.org
Email: admin@papyrus-uk.org

Samaritans
Available 24 hours a day to provide confidential emotional support for people who are experiencing feelings of distress or despair, including those that may lead to suicide.

The Upper Mill
Kingston Road
Ewell
Surrey KT17 2AS
Tel: 08457 90 90 90
www.samaritans.org
Email: jo@samaritans.org

Winston's Wish
Helps bereaved children and young people build their lives after a family death. Offers practical supporting guidance to families, professionals and anyone concerned about a grieving child.

Clara Burgess Centre
Bayshill Road
Cheltenham GL50 8AW
Tel: 0845 20 30 40 5
www.winstonswish.org.uk
Email: info@winstonswish.org.uk

Young Minds

Provides information about the national and local services available to young people.

48–50 St John Street
London EC1M 4DG
Tel: 020 7336 8445
www.youngminds.org.uk
Email: enquiries@youngminds.org.uk

Young NCB (National Children's Bureau)

Free membership network for all children and young people that enables young people to be actively involved in the issues that affect them.

8 Wakley Street
London EC1V 7QE
Tel: 020 7843 6000
www.youngncb.org.uk

Sources of Information about Deliberate Self-harm, Suicide and Mental Health Problems

American Association of Suicidology
5221 Wisconsin Avenue, NW
Washington, DC 20015
USA
Tel: +1 (202) 237 2280
www.suicidology.org
Email: info@suicidology.org

American Foundation for Suicide Prevention
120 Wall Street, 22nd Floor
New York, NY 1005
USA
Tel: +1 (212) 363 3500
www.afsp.org
Email: inquiry@afsp.org

Centre for Suicide Prevention
University of Manchester
Oxford Road
Manchester M13 9PL
www.centre-suicide-prevention.man.ac.uk

Centre for Suicide Research, Oxford

Investigates the causes, treatment and prevention of suicidal behaviour. The programme of work being carried out aims to increase knowledge directly relevant to the prevention of suicide and deliberate self-harm.

University of Oxford
Department of Psychiatry
Warneford Hospital
Oxford OX3 7JX
Tel: 01865 226258
http://cebmh.warne.ox.ac.uk/csr
Email: csr@psychiatry.oxford.ac.uk

International Association for Suicide Prevention

www.med.uio.no/iasp
Email: iasp1960@aol.com

Irish Association of Suicidology

16 New Antrim Street
Castlebar
County Mayo
Ireland
Tel: +353 94 925 0858
www.ias.ie

MIND

National association for mental health.

Granta House
15–19 Broadway
London E15 4BQ
Tel: 0845 766 0163
www.mind.org.uk
Email: contact@mind.org.uk

National Children's Bureau

Undertakes research, evaluation and development projects in order to provide an evidence base that will influence policy and best practice.

8 Wakley Street
London EC1V 7QE
Tel: 020 7843 6000
www.ncb.org.uk

The bureau also has a self-harm specific website:
www.self-harm.org.uk

Trust for the Study of Adolescence
Considers that there is a lack of knowledge and understanding about adolescence
and young adulthood. Aims to close this gap by research, training for professionals
and provision of information for parents, professionals and young people.

23 New Road
Brighton
East Sussex BN1 1WZ
Tel: 01273 693311
www.tsa.uk.com
Email: info@tsa.uk.com

APPENDIX VII
Further Reading

For young people who self-harm and their relatives

Arnold, L. and McGill, A. (1997) *What's the Harm? A Book for Young People who Self-harm or Self-injure.* Bristol: The Basement Project.

This book is written for young people who engage in deliberate self-harm and for friends who are worried about someone who self-harms. It aims to provide information about self-harm, how to stay safe if you engage in self-harm, how to get help and how to help a friend who self-harms.

Arnold, L. and McGill, A. (1998) *The Self-harm Help Book.* Abergavenny: The Basement Project.

This book is written for people who engage in deliberate self-harm. The book aims to show new ways for dealing with feelings of distress and to develop ways of supporting oneself.

Arnold, L. and McGill, A. (2000) *Making Sense of Self-harm.* Abergavenny: The Basement Project.

This book is written for people who want to know more about self-harm and for friends or relatives who are worried about someone who self-harms. It aims to help the reader to understand why people self-harm and to show the reader how he or she can respond helpfully and support someone who self-harms.

Macfarlane, A. and McPherson, A. (1999) *Adolescents: The Agony, the Ecstasy, the Answers – A Book for Parents.* London: Little Brown.

This book shows how parents view their teenagers, and vice versa, in order to enable each to recognise, appreciate and understand the other's viewpoint. It highlights areas of conflict and offers advice on how to get things right.

Based on real questions emailed to the Teenage Health Freak website, the following five books provide health information and advice for teenagers:

Macfarlane, A. and McPherson, A. (2003) *Sex: The Truth (Teenage Health Freak).* Oxford: Oxford University Press.

Macfarlane, A. and McPherson, A. (2004) *Bullying: The Truth (Teenage Health Freak).* Oxford: Oxford University Press.

Macfarlane, A. and McPherson, A. (2004) *Drugs: The Truth (Teenage Health Freak).* Oxford: Oxford University Press.

Macfarlane, A. and McPherson, A. (2004) *Relationships: The Truth (Teenage Health Freak).* Oxford: Oxford University Press.

Macfarlane, A. and McPherson, A. (2005) *Stressed Out (Teenage Health Freak).* Oxford: Oxford University Press.

McPherson, A. and Macfarlane, A. (2002) *Diary of a Teenage Health Freak*, 3rd edn. Oxford: Oxford University Press.

Schmidt, U. and Davidson, K. (2004) *Life After Self-harm*. Brighton: Brunner-Routledge.

This book is written for someone who is in distress and has perhaps self-harmed. It provides a step-by-step guide for the person to navigate through his or her crisis.

For people who have lost someone through suicide

Wertheimer, A. (2001) *A Special Scar: The Experiences of People Bereaved by Suicide*, 2nd edn. Hove: Brunner-Routledge.

This book looks in detail at the stigma surrounding suicide and offers practical help for survivors, relatives and friends of people who have taken their own lives.

For Professionals who work with people who self-harm

Aldridge, D. (1998) *Suicide: The Tragedy of Hopelessness*. London: Jessica Kingsley Publishers.

Drawing on case studies and research, Aldridge constructs a background against which suicidal behaviour can be perceived not as irrational and unpredictable but as an understandable response to social disruption.

Coleman, J. (2004) *Teenage Suicide and Self-harm Training Pack*. Brighton: Trust for the Study of Adolescence.

Based on interviews with young people, parents, friends and workers in the field, this pack offers five sets of training exercises and is accompanied by an audio CD.

Coleman, J. and Schofield, J. (2005) *Key Data on Adolescence, 2005*. Brighton: Trust for the Study of Adolescence.

Provides the latest available information and statistics on young people, covering all aspects of families, health education and crime.

Duffy, D. and Ryan, T. (2004) *New Approaches to Preventing Suicide: A Manual for Practitioners*. London: Jessica Kingsley Publishers.

A useful companion to the government suicide-prevention strategy for England. The contributors offer practical guidance on issues such as risk assessment and management in a range of settings.

Firestone, R.W. (1997) *Suicide and the Inner Voice: Risk Assessment, Treatment and Case Management*. London: Sage Publications.

Firestone believes that the key to understanding suicidal behaviour comes from knowledge of the destructive thought processes of those at risk and an awareness of their origins in family interactions. From an understanding of how one begins a downward spiral of negative internal conversations, professionals can better assess risk and design treatment for depressed and suicidal patients.

Fox, C. and Hawton, K. (2004) *Deliberate Self-Harm in Adolescence*. London: Jessica Kingsley Publishers.

This practical and evidence-based book summarises and evaluates current research into suicidal behaviour. It aims to provide guidance for professionals and parents caring for children and young people at risk of self-harm and suicide.

Hawton, K. and van Heeringen, K. (2000) *The International Handbook of Suicide and Attempted Suicide.* Chichester: John Wiley & Sons.

This handbook brings together, in an easily accessible form, knowledge about the causes of suicidal behaviour and its treatment and prevention.

Levenkron, S. (1998) *Cutting: Understanding and Overcoming Self Mutilation.* New York: W.W. Norton.

Levenkron, a psychotherapist in private practice, takes the reader through the psychological experience of the person who seeks relief from mental anguish in self-inflicted physical pain.

McPherson, A., Donovan, C. and Macfarlane, A. (2002) *Healthcare of Young People: Promotion in Primary Care.* Oxford: Radcliffe Medical Press.

Provides essential practical and useful information to help meet the health needs of adolescents. Useful for GPs, nurses, practice managers and all members of the primary healthcare team.

O'Connor, R. and Sheehy, N. (2000) *Understanding Suicidal Behaviour.* Oxford: BPS Blackwell.

Aims to demystify suicide and shows how regarding it as the product of an insane mind fails to explain why people kill themselves and how those considering suicide may be helped.

Piper, D.E. (2002) *Young People, Suicide and Self-harm.* Brighton: Trust for the Study of Adolescence.

Brings together information from research and clinical practice. Written for those who work with young people who may be suicidal or self-harming.

Shea, S.C. (2002) *The Practical Art of Suicide Assessment: A Guide for Mental Health Professionals and Substance Abuse Counsellors.* Chichester: John Wiley & Sons.

Aims to provide the busy clinician with a no-nonsense set of principles for spotting and assessing suicidal ideation, planning and intent.

Turp, M. (2003) *Hidden Self-harm: Narratives from Pychotherapy.* London: Jessica Kingsley Publishers.

This book is written from a psychoanalytical perspective and draws from a series of case studies, focusing in particular on hidden self-harm.

Van Heeringen, K. (2002) *Understanding Suicidal Behaviour: The Suicidal Process Approach To Research, Treatment and Prevention.* Chichester: John Wiley & Sons.

This book offers a clinical guide to the assessment, treatment and prevention of suicidal behaviour.

Wertheimer, A. (2001) *A Special Scar: The Experiences of People Bereaved by Suicide,* 2nd edn. Hove: Brunner-Routledge.

This book looks in detail at the stigma surrounding suicide and offers practical help for survivors, relatives and friends of people who have taken their own lives.

Yufit, R.I. and Lester, D. (2005) *Assessment, Treatment and Prevention of Suicidal Behaviour.* Chichester: John Wiley & Sons.

This book provides a comprehensive source of information, guidelines and case studies for working with clients at risk of suicide. It offers counsellors, clinicians and other mental health professionals a practical toolbox focusing on screening and assessment, intervention and treatment, and suicide and violence.

For people with a general interest in self-harm

Alvarez, A. (2002) *The Savage God: A Study of Suicide.* London: Bloomsbury.

This book explores the cultural attitudes, theories, truths and fallacies surrounding suicide from the perspective of literature.

Fox, C. and Hawton, K. (2004) *Deliberate Self-Harm in Adolescence.* London: Jessica Kingsley Publishers.

This practical and evidence-based book summarises and evaluates current research into suicidal behaviour. It aims to provide guidance for professionals and parents caring for children and young people at risk of self-harm and suicide.

Hill, K. (1995) *The Long Sleep: Young People and Suicide.* London: Virago.

This book explores the origins, symptoms and meanings of young peoples' suicidal crises. Combining moving accounts from relatives and young attempters with the evidence of extensive research into the subject, this book offers important and timely insights into an area fraught with fear and denial.

Redfield Jamison, K. (1999) *Night Falls Fast: Understanding Suicide.* London: Picador.

This book, which is based strongly on research, traces the network of reasons underlying suicide and aims to provide a better understanding of the suicidal mind and a chance to recognise the person at risk.

Turp, M. (2003) *Hidden Self-harm: Narratives from Psychotherapy.* London: Jessica Kingsley Publishers.

This book is written from a psychoanalytical perspective and draws from a series of case studies, focusing in particular on hidden self-harm.

References

Adams, J. and Adams, M. (1996) The association among negative life events, perceived problem-solving alternatives, depression and suicidal ideation in adolescent psychiatric patients. *Journal of Child Psychiatry and Psychology 37*, 715–720.

Adams, M. and Adams, J. (1991) Life events, depression and perceived problem-solving alternatives in adolescents. *Journal of Child Psychology and Psychiatry 32*, 811–820.

Allgulander, C. (2000) Psychiatric aspects of suicidal behaviour: anxiety disorders. In K. Hawton and K. van Heeringen (eds) *The International Handbook of Suicide and Attempted Suicide*. Chichester: John Wiley & Sons.

Allison, S., Pearce, C., Martin, G., Miller, K. and Long, R. (1995) Parental influence, pessimism and adolescent suicidality. *Archives of Suicide Research 1*, 229–242.

Alty, A. and Rodham, K. (1998) The ouch factor! Problems in conducting sensitive research. *Qualitative Health Research 8*, 275–282.

American Academy of Child and Adolescent Psychiatry (2001) Practice parameter for the assessment and treatment of children and adolescents with suicidal behaviour. *Journal of the American Academy of Child and Adolescent Psychiatry 40 (Suppl.)*, 24S–51S.

American Foundation for Suicide Prevention, American Association of Suicidology and Annenberg Public Policy Center (2001) Reporting on suicide: guidelines for the media. www.afsp.org/education/recommendations/1/index.html. Accessed 24 August 2005.

American Psychiatric Association (1980) *Diagnostic and Statistical Manual of Mental Disorders*. Washington, DC: American Psychiatric Association.

Anderman, C., Cheadle, A., Curry, S., Diehr, P., Shultz, L. and Wagner, E. (1995) Selection bias related to parental consent in school-based survey research. *Evaluation Review 19*, 663–674.

Andrews, J.A. and Lewinsohn, P.M. (1992) Suicidal attempts among older adolescents: prevalence and co-occurrence with psychiatric disorders. *Journal of the American Academy of Child and Adolescent Psychiatry 31*, 655–662.

Appleby, L., Amos, T., Doyle, U., Tomenson, B. and Woodman, M. (1996) General practitioners and young suicides. *British Journal of Psychiatry 168*, 330–333.

Apter, A., Plutchik, R. and Van Praag, H.M. (1993) Anxiety, impulsivity and depressed mood in relation to suicidal and violent behaviour. *Acta Psychiatrica Scandinavica 87*, 1–5.

Aquilano, W.S. and Loscuito, L.A. (1990) Effects of interview mode on self-reported drug use. *Pubic Opinion Quarterly 54*, 362–395.

Aresman, E., Townsend, E., Hawton, K., Bremmer, S., Feldman, E., Goldney, R., *et al* (2001) Psychosocial and pharmacological treatment of patients following deliberate self-harm: the methodological issues involved in evaluating effectiveness. *Suicide and Life-Threatening Behavior 31*, 196–180.

Arnett, J. (1991) Heavy metal and reckless behaviour among adolescents. *Journal of Youth and Adolescence 20*, 573–592.

Arnold, L. and McGill, A. (1998) *The Self-Harm Help Book*. Abergavenny: The Basement Project.

Australasian College for Emergency Medicine and the Royal Australian and New Zealand College of Psychiatrists (2000) *Guidelines for the Management of Deliberate Self-harm in Young People*. Melbourne: Australian College for Emergency Medicine and the Royal Australian and New Zealand College of Psychiatrists.

Bagley, C. (1992) Development of an adolescent stress scale for use by school counsellors. *School Psychology International 13*, 31–49.

Bagley, C. and Tremblay, P. (2000) Elevated rates of suicidal behavior in gay, lesbian, and bisexual youth. *Crisis 21*, 111–117.

Bancroft, J., Hawton, K., Simkin, S., Kingston, B., Cumming, C. and Whitwell, D. (1979) The reasons people give for taking overdoses: a further enquiry. *British Journal of Medical Psychology 52*, 353–365.

Bancroft, J., Skrimshire, A.M. and Simkin, S. (1976) The reasons people give for taking overdoses. *British Journal of Psychiatry 128*, 538–548.

Bargh, J.A., McKenna, K.Y.A., and Fitzsimons, G.M. (2002) Can you see the real me? Activation and expression of the true self on the Internet. *Journal of Social Issues 58*, 33–48.

Barnes, M.D., Penrod, C., Neiger, B.L., Merrill, R.M., Thackeray, R. and Eggett, D.L. (2003) Measuring the relevance of evaluation criteria among health information seekers on the Internet. *Journal of Health Psychology 8*, 71–82.

Batt, A., Eudier, F., Phillippe, A. and Pommereau, X. (2001) Suicidal behaviour in France. In A. Schmidtke, U. Bille-Brahe, D. De Leo and A. Kerkhof (eds) *Suicidal Behaviour in Europe*. Göttingen: Hogrefe and Huber.

Bauerle Bass, S. (2003) How will Internet use affect the patient? A review of computer network and closed Internet-based system studies and the implications in understanding how the use of the Internet affects patient populations. *Journal of Health Psychology 8*, 25–38.

Beautrais, A. (2003) Suicide in New Zealand. I: time trends and epidemiology. *New Zealand Medical Journal 116*, 460–471.

Beautrais, A.L., Joyce, P.R. and Mulder, R.T. (1997) Precipitating factors and life events in serious suicide attempts among youths aged 13 through 24 years. *Journal of American Academy of Child and Adolescent Psychiatry 36*, 1543–1551.

Beautrais, A.L., Joyce, P.R., Mulder, R.T., Fergusson, D.M., Deavoll, B.J. and Nightingale, S.K. (1996) Prevalence and comorbidity of mental disorders in persons making serious suicide attempts: a case control study. *American Journal of Psychiatry 153*, 1009–1014.

Beck, A.T. (1967) *Depression: Clinical, Experimental and Theoretical Aspects*. New York: Harper & Row. Beck, A.T., Beck, R. and Kovacs, M. (1975) Classification of suicidal behaviours: I. Quantifying intent and medical lethality. *American Journal of Psychiatry 132*, 285–287.

Beck, A.T., Schuyler, D. and Herman, I. (1974) Development of suicidal intent scales. In A.T. Beck, H.L.P. Resnick and D. Lettieri (eds) *The Prediction of Suicide*. Bowie, MD: Charles Press.

Beebe, T.J., Harnson, P.A., McRae, J.A., Anderson, R.E. and Fullerson, J.A. (1998) An evaluation of computer assisted self-interviews in a school setting. *Public Opinion Quarterly 62*, 623–632.

Bennewith, O., Gunnell, D., Peters, T.J., Hawton, K. and House, A. (2004) Variations in the hospital management of self-harm in adults in England: observational study. *British Medical Journal 328*, 1108–1109.

Bennewith, O., Stocks, N., Gunnell, D., Peters, T.J., Evans, M.O. and Sharp, D.J. (2002) General practice based intervention to prevent repeat episodes of deliberate self-harm: cluster randomised controlled trial. *British Medical Journal 324*, 1254–1260.

Bensley, L.S., Van Eenwyk, J., Spieker, S.J. and Schoder, M.N. (1999) Self-reported abuse history and adolescent problem behaviours. I: antisocial and suicidal behaviours. *Journal of Adolescent Health 24*, 163–172.

Benson, M.D. and Torpy, E.J. (1995) Sexual behavior in junior high school students. *Obstetrics and Gynaecology 85*, 279–284.

Bhugra, D., Desai, M. and Baldwin, D.S. (1999) Attempted suicide in west London. I: rates across ethnic communities. *Psychological Medicine 29*, 1125–1130.

Bhugra, D., Thompson, N., Singh, J. and Fellow-Smith, E. (2003) Inception rates of deliberate self-harm among adolescents in west London. *International Journal of Social Psychiatry 49*, 247–250.

Bjarnason, T. and Thorlindsson, T. (1994) Manifest predictors of past suicide attempts in a population of Icelandic adolescents. *Suicide and Life-Threatening Behavior 24*, 350–358.

Boergers, J., Spirito, A., and Donaldson, D. (1998) Reasons for adolescent suicide attempts: associations with psychosocial functioning. *Journal of the American Academy of Child and Adolescent Psychiatry 37*, 1287–1293.

Bond, L., Carlin, J.B., Thomas, L., Robyn, K. and Patton, G. (2001) Does bullying cause emotional problems? A prospective study of young teenagers. *British Medical Journal 323*, 480–484.

Boreham, R. and Blenkinsop, S. (2004) *Drug Use, Smoking and Drinking Among Young People in England in 2003*. London: The Stationery Office.

Brain, K.L., Haines, J. and Williams, C.L. (1998) The psychophysiology of self mutilation: evidence of tension reduction. *Archives of Suicide Research 4*, 227–242.

Brent, D.A., Perper, J. and Allman, C. (1987) Alcohol, firearms and suicide among youth: temporal trends in Allegheny County, PA, 1960–1983. *Journal of the American Medical Association 257*, 3369–3372.

Brent, D.A., Perper, J., Moritz, G., Allman, C., Friend, A., Roth, C., *et al.* (1993) Psychiatric risk factors for adolescent suicide: a case control study. *Journal of the American Academy of Child and Adolescent Psychiatry 32*, 521–529.

Brent, D.A., Johnson, B.A., Perper, J., Connelly, J., Bridge, J., Bartle, S. and Rather, C. (1994) Personality disorder, personality traits, impulsive violence and completed suicide in adolescents. *Journal of the American Academy of Child and Adolescent Psychiatry 33*, 1080–1086.

Brent, D.A., Bridge, J., Johnson, B. and Connelly, J. (1996) Suicidal behaviour runs in families: A controlled family study of adolescent suicide victims. *Archives of General Psychiatry 53*, 1145–1149.

Brindis, C., Wolfe, A.L., McCarter, V., Ball, S. and Starbuck, M.S. (1995). The associations between immigrant status and risk-behavior patterns in Latino adolescents. *Journal of Adolescent Health 17*, 99–105.

British Educational Research Association (1992) *Ethical Guidelines for Educational Research.* Nottingham: British Educational Research Association.

Brown, G.K., Have, T.T., Henriques, G.R., Xie, S.X., Hollander, J.E. and Beck, A.T. (2005) Cognitive therapy for the prevention of suicide attempts: a randomized controlled trial. *Journal of the American Medical Association 294*, 563–570.

Browne, K.D. and Hamilton-Giachritsis, C. (2005) The influence of violent media on children and adolescents: a public health approach. *Lancet 365*, 702–710.

Browne, K., Henriques, G.R., Sosdjan, D. and Beck, A.T. (2004) Suicide intent and accurate expectations of lethality: predictors of medical lethality of suicide attempts. *Journal of Consulting and Clinical Psychology 72*, 1170–1174.

Buglass, D. and Horton, H.J. (1974) A scale for predicting subsequent suicidal behaviour. *British Journal of Psychiatry 124*, 573–578.

Burgess, S., Hawton, K. and Loveday, G. (1998) Adolescents who take overdoses: outcome in terms of changes in psychopathology and the adolescents' attitudes to their care and to their overdoses. *Journal of Adolescence 21*, 209–218.

Cantor, C.H. (2000) Suicide in the Western world. In K. Hawton and K. van Heeringen (eds) *The International Handbook of Suicide and Attempted Suicide*. Chichester: John Wiley & Sons.

Carlton, P.A. and Deane, F.P. (2000) Impact of attitudes and suicidal ideation on adolescents' intentions to seek professional psychological help. *Journal of Adolescence 23*, 33–45.

Carver, C.S., Pozo, C., Harris, S.D., Noriega, V., Scheier, M.F., Robinson, D.S., *et al.* (1993) How coping mediates the effect of optimism on distress: a study of women with early stage breast cancer. *Journal of Personality and Social Psychology 65*, 375–390.

Catalan, J. (2000) Sexuality, reproductive cycle and suicidal behaviour. In K. Hawton and K. Van Heeringen (eds) *The International Handbook of Suicide and Attempted Suicide*. Chichester: John Wiley & Sons.

Centers for Disease Control and Prevention (2004) Youth risk behavior surveillance - United States, 2003. *Morbidity and Mortality Weekly Report 53*.

Chandy, J.M., Blum, R.W.W. and Resnick, M.D. (1996) History of sexual abuse and parental alcohol misuse: risk, outcomes and protective factors in adolescents. *Child and Adolescent Social Work Journal 13*, 411–432.

Choquet, M. and Ledoux, S. (1994) *Adolescents: enqute nationale*. Paris: INSERM.

Choquet, M. and Menke, H. (1989) Suicidal thoughts during early adolescence: prevalence, associated troubles and help-seeking behavior. *Acta Psychiatrica Scandinavica 81*, 170–177.

Choquet, M., Darves-Bornoz, J.-M., Ledoux, S., Manfredi, R. and Hassler, C. (1997) Self-reported health and behavioral problems among adolescent victims of rape in France: results of a cross-sectional survey. *Child Abuse and Neglect 21*, 823–832.

Choquet, M., Facy, F. and Davidson, F. (1980) Suicide and attempted suicide among adolescents in France. In R.D.T. Farmer and S. Hirsch (eds) *The Suicide Syndrome*. London: Cambridge University Press.

Clarke, G.N., Hawkins, W., Murphy, M. and Sheeber, L. (1993) School-based primary prevention of depressive symptomatology in adolescents: findings from two studies. *Journal of Adolescent Research 8*, 183–204.

Cohen, S. and Wills, T.A. (1985) Stress, social support and the buffering hypothesis. *Psychological Bulletin 98*, 310–357.

Cole, D.A. (1989) Psychopathology of adolescent suicide: hopelessness, coping beliefs and depression. *Journal of Abnormal Psychology 98*, 248–255.

Coll, X., Law, F., Tobias, A., Hawton, K. and Tomàs, J. (2001) Abuse and deliberate self-poisoning in women: a matched case-control study. *Child Abuse and Neglect 25*, 1291–1302.

Collishaw, S., Maughan, B., Goodman, R. and Pickles, A. (2004) Time trends in adolescent well-being. *Journal of Child Psychology and Psychiatry 45*, 1350–1362.

Conrad, N. (1992) Stress and knowledge of suicidal others as factors in suicidal behavior of high school adolescents. *Issues in Mental Health Nursing 13*, 95–104.

Corcoran, P., Keeley, H.S., O'Sullivan, M. and Perry, I.J. (2004) The incidence and repetition of attempted suicide in Ireland. *European Journal of Public Health 14*, 19–23.

Cotgrove, A.J., Zirinsky, L., Black, D. and Weston, D. (1995) Secondary prevention of attempted suicide in adolescence. *Journal of Adolescence 18*, 569–577.

Darves-Bornoz, J.M., Choquet, M., Ledoux, S., Gasquet, I. and Manfredi, R. (1998) Gender differences in symptoms of adolescents reporting sexual assault. *Social Psychiatry and Psychiatric Epidemiology 33*, 111–117.

Davis, J.M. and Sandovel, J. (1991) *Suicidal Youth: School-Based Intervention and Prevention.* San Francisco: Jossey Bass.

Davis, J.M., Sandoval, J. and Wilson, M.P. (1988) Strategies for the primary prevention of adolescent suicide. *School Psychology Review 17*, 559–569.

De Anda, D. and Smith, M.A. (1993) Differences among adolescent, young adult and adult callers to suicide help-lines. *Social Work 38*, 421–428.

De Leo, D. and Heller, T.S. (2004) Who are the kids who self-harm? An Australian self-report school survey. *Medical Journal of Australia 181*, 140–144.

De Wilde, E.J. (2000) Adolescent suicidal behaviour: a general population perspective. In K. Hawton and K. Van Hereringen (eds) *The International Handbook of Suicide and Attempted Suicide.* Chichester: John Wiley & Sons.

Dent, C.W., Galaif, J., Sussman, S., Stacey, A., Burton, D. and Fley, B. R. (1993) Demographic, psychosocial and behavioural differences in samples of actively and passively consented adolescents. *Addictive Behaviours 18*, 51–56.

Department of Health (2004) *National Service Framework for Children, Young People and Maternity Service: Care Standards.* London: Department of Health.

Dinges, N.G. and Duong-Tran, Q. (1994) Suicide ideation and suicide attempts among American Indian and Alaska native boarding school adolescents. *American Indian and Alaskan Native Mental Health Research Monograph Series 4*, 168–188.

Domènech, E., Canals, J. and Fernández-Ballart, J. (1992) Suicidal ideation among Spanish schoolchildren: a three-year follow-up study of a pubertal population. *Personality and Individual Differences 13*, 1055–1057.

Dubow, E.F., Kausch, D.F., Blum, M.C., Reed, J. and Bush, E. (1989) Correlates of suicidal ideation and attempts in a community sample of junior high and high school students. *Journal of Clinical Child Psychology 18*, 158–166.

Edman, J.L., Andrade, N.N., Gilpa, J., Foster, J., Danko, G.P., Yates, A., *et al.* (1998) Depressive symptoms among Filipino American adolescents. *Cultural Diversity and Mental Health 4*, 45–54.

Embree, B.G. and Whitehead, P.C. (1993) Validity and reliability of self-reported drinking behaviour: dealing with the problem of response bias. *Journal of Studies on Alcohol 54*, 334–344.

Eng, T.R (2001) *The eHealth Landscape: A Terrain Map of Emerging Information and Communication Technologies in Health and Health Care.* Princeton, NJ: The Robert Wood Johnson Foundation.

Eskin, M. (1995) Suicidal behavior as related to social support and assertiveness among Swedish and Turkish high school students: a cross-cultural investigation. *Journal of Clinical Psychology, 51*, 158–172.

Esters, I.G., Cooker, P.G. and Ittenbach, R.F. (1998) Effects of a unit of instruction in mental health on rural adolescents' conceptions of mental illness and attitudes about seeking help. *Adolescence 33*, 469–476.

Evans, E., Hawton, K. and Rodham, K. (2004) Factors associated with suicidal phenomena in adolescents: a systematic review of population-based studies. *Clinical Psychology Review 24,* 957–979.

Evans, E., Hawton, K., Rodham, K. and Deeks, J. (2005a) The prevalence of suicidal phenomena in adolescents: a systematic review of population-based studies. *Suicide and Life-Threatening Behavior 35,* 239–250.

Evans, E., Hawton, K. and Rodham, K. (2005b) In what ways are adolescents who engage in self-harm or experience thoughts of self-harm different in terms of help-seeking, communication and coping strategies? *Journal of Adolescence 28,* 573–587.

Evans, J., Evans, M., Morgan, H.G., Hayward, A. and Gunnell, D. (2005) Crisis card following self-harm: 12 month follow-up of a randomised controlled trial. *British Journal of Psychiatry 187,* 186–187.

Evans, M.O., Morgan, H.G., Hayward, A. and Gunnell, D.J. (1999) Crisis telephone consultation for deliberate self-harm patients: effects on repetition. *British Journal of Psychiatry 175,* 23–27.

Evans, W., Smith, M., Hill, G., Albers, E. and Neufeld, J. (1996) Rural adolescent views of risk and protective factors associated with suicide. *Crisis Intervention 3,* 1–12.

Favazza, A.R. and Conterio, K. (1989) Female habitual self-mutilators. *Acta Psychiatrica Scandinavica 79,* 283–289.

Fekete, S., Schmidtke, A., Etzersdorfer, E. and Gailiene, D. (1998) Media reports in Hungary, Austria, Germany and Lithuania in 1981 and 1991: reflection, mediation and changes of sociocultural attitudes towards suicide in the mass media. In D. De Leo, A. Schmidtke and R.F.W. Diekstra (eds) *Suicide Prevention: A Holistic Approach.* Dordrecht: Kluwer.

Fekete, S., Voros, V. and Osvath, P. (2004) Suicidal behaviour and psychopathology in adolescents: results of a self-report survey among 15- and 16-year old adolescent people in Hungary. *European Neuropsychopharmacology 14,* S365–S365.

Ferguson, T. (1998) Digital doctoring: opportunities and challenges in electronic patient-physician communication. *Journal of the American Medical Association 280,* 1261–1262.

Fergusson, D.M. and Lynskey, M.T. (1995) Childhood circumstances, adolescent adjustment and suicide attempts in a New Zealand birth cohort. *Journal of the American Academy of Child and Adolescent Psychiatry 34,* 612–622.

Fergusson, D.M., Horwood, L.J., Ridder, E.M. and Beautrais, A.L. (2005a) Sexual orientation and mental health in a birth cohort of young adults. *Psychological Medicine 35,* 971–981.

Fergusson, D.M., Horwood, L.J., Ridder, E.M. and Beautrais, A.L (2005b) Suicidal behaviour in adolescence and subsequent mental health outcomes in young adulthood. *Psychological Medicine 35,* 983–993.

Finlay, F. (1998) Providing healthcare information suitable for adolescents. *Health Visitor 71,* 16–18.

Flisher, A.J., Kramer, R.A., Hoven, C.W., Greenwald, S., Alegria, M., Bird, H.R., *et al.* (1997) Psychosocial characteristics of physically abused children and adolescents. *Journal of American Academy of Child and Adolescent Psychiatry 36,* 123–131.

Fombonne, E. (1995) Depressive disorders: time trends and possible explanatory mechanisms. In M. Rutter and D.J. Smith (eds) *Psychosocial Disorders in Young People: Time Trends and Their Causes.* Chichester: John Wiley & Sons.

Fornaciari, C. and Roca, M. (1999) The age of clutter: conducting effective research using the Internet. *Journal of Management Education 23,* 732–742.

Fortune, S., Sinclair, J. and Hawton, K. (submitted for publication) Adolescents' views on preventing self-harm: a large community study.

Fox, C. and Hawton, K. (2004) *Deliberate Self-harm in Adolescence.* London: Jessica Kingsley Publishers.

Galaif, E.R., Chou, C.P., Sussman, S. and Dent, C.W. (1998) Depression, suicidal ideation and substance use among continuation high school students. *Journal of Youth and Adolescence 27,* 405–429.

Ganster, D.C. and Victor, B. (1988) The impact of social support on mental and physical health. *British Journal of Medical Psychology 61,* 17–36.

Garfinkel, B.D. (1989) The components of school-based suicide prevention. *Residential Treatment for Children and Youth 7,* 97–116.

Garland, A. Shaffer, D. and Whittle, B. (1989) A national survey of school-based adolescent suicide prevention programs. *Journal of the American Academy of Child and Adolescent Psychiatry 28,* 931–934.

Garner, H.G. (1975) An adolescent suicide, the mass media and the educator. *Adolescence 10,* 241–246.

Garrison, C.Z., Addy, C.L., Jackson, K.L., McKeown, R.E. and Waller, J.L. (1991) A longitudinal study of suicidal ideation in young adolescents. *Journal of the American Academy of Child and Adolescent Psychiatry 30,* 597–603.

Gartrell, J.W., Jarvis, G.K. and Derksen, L. (1993) Suicidality among adolescent Alberta Indians. *Suicide and Life-Threatening Behavior 23,* 366–373.

Goldacre, M. and Hawton, K. (1985) Repetition of self-poisoning and subsequent death in adolescents who take overdoses. *British Journal of Psychiatry 146,* 486–489.

Gould, M.S. and Davidson, L. (1988) Suicide contagion among adolescents. In A.R. Stiffman and R.A. Feldman (eds) *Advances in Adolescent Mental Health.* Greenwich, CT: JAI Press.

Gould, M., Greenberg, T., Velting, D. and Shaffer, D. (2003) Youth suicide risk and preventive interventions: areview of the past 10 years. *Journal of the American Academy of Child and Adolescent Psychiatry 42,* 386–405.

Gould, M., Munfakh, J.L.H., Lubell, K., Kleinman, M. and Parker, S. (2002) Seeking help from the Internet during adolescence. *Journal of the American Academy of Child and Adolescent Psychiatry 41,* 1182–1189.

Gould, M.S., Petrie, K., Kleinman, M.H. and Wallenstein, S. (1994) Clustering of attempted suicide: New Zealand national data. *International Journal of Epidemiology 23,* 1185–1189.

Gould, M.S., Velting, D., Kleinman, M., Lucas, C., Thomas, J.G. and Chung, M. (2004) Teenagers' attitudes about coping strategies and help-seeking behaviour. *Journal of the American Academy of Child and Adolescent Psychiatry 43,* 1124–1133.

Gould, M.S., Wallenstein, S. and Davidson, L. (1989) Suicide clusters: a critical review. *Suicide and Life-Threatening Behavior 19,* 17–29.

Gratz, K.L. (2003) Risk factors for and functions of deliberate self-harm: an empirical and conceptual review. *Clinical Psychology: Science and Practice 10,* 192–205.

Griffiths, M. (2002) Using the Internet for qualitative clinical research. *Clinical Psychology 10,* 27–30.

Grossman, D.C., Milligan, B.C. and Deyo, R.A. (1991) Risk factors for suicide attempts among Navajo adolescents. *American Journal of Public Health 81,* 870–874.

Grootenhuis, M., Hawton, K., van Rooijen, L. and Fagg, J. (1994) Attempted suicide in Oxford and Utrecht. *British Journal of Psychiatry 165,* 73–78.

Gunnell, D., Bennewith, O., Peters, T.J., House, A. and Hawton, K. (2005) The epidemiology and management of self-harm amongst adults in England. *Journal of Public Health 27,* 67–73.

Guthrie, E., Kapur, N., Mackway-Jones, K., Chew-Graham, C., Moorey, J., Mendel, E., *et al.* (2001) Randomised controlled trial of brief psychological intervention after deliberate self-poisoning. *British Medical Journal 323*, 135–137.

Happell, B., Summers, M. and Pinikahana, J. (2003) Measuring the effectiveness of the national Mental Health Triage Scale in an emergency department. *International Journal of Mental Health Nursing 12*, 288–292.

Harrington, R. (2001) Depression, suicide and deliberate self-harm in adolescence. *British Medical Bulletin 57*, 47–60.

Harrington, R., Kerfoot, M., Dyer, E., McNiven, F., Gill, J., Harrington, V., *et al.* (1998a) Randomised trial of a home-based family intervention for children who have deliberately poisoned themselves. *Journal of the American Academy of Child and Adolescent Psychiatry 37*, 512–518.

Harrington, R., Whittaker, J., Shoebridge, P. and Campbell, F. (1998b) Systematic reviews of efficacy of cognitive behaviour therapies in childhood and adolescent depressive disorders. *British Medical Journal 316*, 1559–1563.

Harriss, L. and Hawton, K. (2005) Suicidal intent in deliberate self-harm and the risk of suicide: the predictive power of the Suicide Intent Scale. *Journal of Affective Disorders 86*, 225–233.

Harriss, L., Hawton, K. and Zahl, D. (2005) The value of measuring suicidal intent in the assessment of deliberate self-harm patients. *British Journal of Psychiatry 186*, 60–66.

Hawton, K. (1990) Self-cutting: can it be prevented? In K. Hawton and P. Cowen (eds) *Dilemmas and Difficulties in the Management of Psychiatric Patients.* Oxford: Oxford University Press.

Hawton, K. (1992) By their own young hand. *British Medical Journal, 304*, 1000.

Hawton, K. and Blackstock, E. (1976) General practice aspects of self-poisoning and self-injury. *Psychological Medicine 6*, 571–575.

Hawton, K. and Catalan, J. (1987) *Attempted Suicide: A Practical Guide to its Nature and Management.* Oxford: Oxford University Press.

Hawton, K. and Fagg, J. (1998) Suicide and other causes of death following attempted suicide. *British Journal of Psychiatry, 152*, 259–266.

Hawton, K. and Fagg, J. (1992) Trends in deliberate self-poisoning and self-injury in adolescents: a study of characteristics and trends in Oxford, 1976–1989. *British Journal of Psychiatry 161*, 816–823.

Hawton, K. and Goldacre, M. (1982) Hospital admissions for adverse effects of medicinal agents (mainly self-poisoning) among adolescents in the Oxford region. *British Journal of Psychiatry 141*, 106–170.

Hawton, K. and Harriss, L. (submitted for publication) Deliberate self-harm in young people: characteristics and subsequent mortality in a 20 year cohort.

Hawton, K. and Kirk, J. (1989) Problem solving. In K. Hawton, P. Salkovskis, J. Kirk and D.M. Clark (eds) *Cognitive Behaviour Therapy for Psychiatric Problems: A Practical Guide.* Oxford: Oxford University Press.

Hawton, K. and Williams, K. (2001) The connection between media and suicidal behaviour warrants serious attention. *Crisis 22*, 137–140.

Hawton, K. and Williams, K. (2002) Influences of the media on suicide: researchers, policy makers, and media personnel need to collaborate on guidelines. *British Medical Journal 325*, 1374–1375.

Hawton, K., Arensman, E., Townsend, E., Bremner, S., Feldman, E., Goldney, R., *et al.* (1998) Deliberate self-harm: a systematic review of the efficacy of psychosocial and pharmacological treatments in preventing repetition. *British Medical Journal 317*, 441–447.

Hawton, K., Casey, D., Simkin, S., Bale, E., and Shepherd, A. (2003a) *Deliberate Self-harm in Oxford, 2003*. Oxford: Centre for Suicide Research, University of Oxford.

Hawton, K., Cole, D., O'Grady, J. and Osborn, M. (1982a) Motivational aspects of deliberate self-poisoning in adolescents. *British Journal of Psychiatry 141*, 286–291.

Hawton, K., Fagg, J. and Simkin, S. (1996) Deliberate self-poisoning and self-injury in children and adolescents under the age of 16 years in Oxford, 1976–1993. *British Journal of Psychiatry 169*, 202–208.

Hawton, K., Fagg, J., Simkin, S., Bale, E. and Bond, A. (1997) Trends in deliberate self-harm in Oxford 1985-1995: implications for clinical services and the prevention of suicide. *British Journal of Psychiatry 171*, 556–560.

Hawton, K., Hall, S., Simkin, S., Bale, E., Bond, A., Codd, S. and Stewart, A. (2003b) Deliberate self-harm in adolescents: a study of characteristics and trends in Oxford, 1999–2000. *Journal of Child Psychology and Psychiatry 44*, 1191–1198.

Hawton, K., Harriss, L., Hall, S., Simkin, S., Bale, E. and Bond, A. (2003c) Deliberate self-harm in Oxford, 1990–2000: a time of change in patient characteristics. *Psychological Medicine 33*, 987–996.

Hawton, K., Harriss, L., Hodder, K., Simkin, S., and Gunnell, D. (2001) The influence of the economic and social environment on deliberate self-harm and suicide: an ecological and person-based study. *Psychological Medicine 31*, 827–836.

Hawton, K., Harriss, L., Simkin, S., Bale, E. and Bond, A. (2004a) Self-cutting: patient characteristics compared with self-poisoners. *Suicide and Life-Threatening Behavior 34*, 199–208.

Hawton, K., Houston, K. and Shepperd, R. (1999a) Suicide in young people: study of 174 cases, aged under 25 years, based on coroners and medical records. *British Journal of Psychiatry 175*, 271–276.

Hawton, K., Kingsbury, S., Steinhardt, K., James, A. and Fagg, J. (1999b) Repetition of deliberate self-harm by adolescents: the role of psychological factors. *Journal of Adolescence 22*, 369–378.

Hawton, K., O'Grady, J., Osborn, M. and Cole, D. (1982b) Adolescents who take overdoses: their characteristics, problems and contacts with helping agencies. *British Journal of Psychiatry 140*, 118–123.

Hawton, K., Osborn, M., OGrady, J. and Cole, D. (1982c) Classification of adolescents who take overdoses. *British Journal of Psychiatry 140*, 124–132.

Hawton, K., Rodham, K., Evans, E. and Harriss, L. (submitted for publication) Adolescents who self-harm: a comparison of those who present to the general hospital and those who do not.

Hawton, K., Rodham, K., Evans, E. and Weatherall, R. (2002) Deliberate self-harm in adolescents: self-report survey in schools in England. *British Medical Journal 325*, 1207–1211.

Hawton, K., Simkin, S., Deeks, J., Cooper, J., Johnston, A., Walters, K. *et al.* 2004b) UK legislation on analgesic packs: before and after study of long term effect on poisonings. *British Medical Journal 329*, 1076–1079.

Hawton, K., Simkin, S., Deeks, J.J., O'Connor, S., Keen, A., Altman, D.G., *et al.* (1999c) Effects of a drug overdose in a television drama on presentations to hospital for self-poisoning: time series and questionnaire study. *British Medical Journal 318*, 972–977.

Hawton, K., Zahl, D. and Weatherall, R. (2003d). Suicide following self-harm: long term follow-up of patients who presented to a general hospital. *British Journal of Psychiatry 182*, 537–542.

Hazell, P. (1991) Postvention after teenage suicide: an Australian experience. *Journal of Adolescence 14*, 335–342.

Hazell, P. and King, R. (1996) Arguments for and against teaching suicide prevention in schools. *Australian and New Zealand Journal of Psychiatry 30*, 633–642.

Headlam, H.K., Goldsmith, R.J., Hanenson, I.B. and Raul, J.L. (1979) Demographic characteristics of adolescents with self-poisoning: survey of 235 instances in Cincinnati, Ohio. *Clinical Pediatrics 18*, 147.

Heled, E. and Read, J. (2005) Young people's opinions about the causes of, and solutions to, New Zealand's high youth suicide rate. *Suicide and Life-Threatening Behavior 35*, 170–180.

Hennig, C.W., Crabtree, C.R. and Baum, D. (1998) Mental health CPR: peer contracting as a response to potential suicide in adolescents. *Archives of Suicide Research 4*, 169–187.

Herrell, R., Goldberg, J., William, R.T., Ramakrishnan, V., Lyons, M., Eissen, S. and Tsuang, M.T. (1999) Sexual orientation and suicidality. *Archives of General Psychiatry 56*, 867–874.

Heslop, L., Elsom, S. and Parker, N. (2000) Improving continuity of care across psychiatric and emergency services: combining patient data within a participatory action research framework. *Journal of Advanced Nursing 31*, 135–143.

Hill, K. (1995) *The Long Sleep: Young People and Suicide*. London: Virago.

Hjelmeland, H., Hawton, K., Nordvik, H., Bille-Brahe, U., De Leo, D., Fekete, S., *et al.* (2002) Why people engage in parasuicide: a cross cultural study of intentions. *Suicide and Life-Threatening Behavior 32*, 380–394.

HMSO (1989) *Children's Act 1989*. London: The Stationery Office.

Hopkins, C. (2002) But what about the really ill, poorly people? An ethnographic study into what it means to nurses on medical admissions units to have people who have harmed themselves as their patients. *Journal of Psychiatric and Mental Health Nursing 9*, 147–154.

Horrocks, J., Price, S., House, A. and Owens, D. (2003) Self injury attendances in the accident and emergency department: clinical database study. *British Journal of Psychiatry 183*, 34–39.

Houston, K., Hawton, K. and Shepperd, R. (2001) Suicide in young people aged 15–24: a psychological autopsy study. *Journal of Affective Disorders 63*, 159–170.

Hovey, J.D. and King, L.A. (1996) Acculturative stress, depression and suicidal ideation among immigrant and second generation Latino adolescents. *Journal of the American Academy of Child and Adolescent Psychiatry 35*, 1183–1192.

Hultén, A., Jiang, G.X., Wasserman, D., Hawton, K., Hjelmeland, H., De Leo, D., *et al.* (2001) Repetition of attempted suicide among teenagers in Europe: frequency, timing and risk factors. *European Child and Adolescent Psychiatry 10*, 161–169.

James, D. and Hawton, K. (1985) Overdoses: explanations and attitudes of significant others. *British Journal of Pscyhiatry 146*, 481–485.

Jobes, D.A., Berman, A.L. and O'Caroll, P.W. (1996) The Kurt Cobain suicide crisis: perspectives from research, public health and the news media. *Suicide and Life-Threatening Behavior 26*, 260–269.

Joffe, R.T., Offord, D.R. and Boyle, M.H. (1988) Ontario child health study: suicidal behavior in youth age 12–16 years. *American Journal of Psychiatry 145*, 1420–1423.

Juon, H.-S., Nam, J.J. and Ensminger, M.E. (1994) Epidemiology of suicidal behavior among Korean adolescents. *Journal of Child Psychology and Psychiatry and Allied Disciplines 35*, 663–676.

Kalafat, J. and Elias, M. (1994) An evaluation of a school-based suicide awareness intervention. *Suicide and Life-Threatening Behavior 24*, 224–233.

Kalafat, J. and Elias, M. (1995) Suicide prevention in an educational context: broad and narrow foci. *Suicide and Life-Threatening Behavior 25*, 123–133.

Kalafat, J. and Gigliano, C. (1996) The use of simulations to assess the impact of an adolescent suicide response curriculum. *Suicide and Life-Threatening Behavior 26*, 359–364.

Kaltiala-Heino, R., Rimpela, M., Marttunen, M., Rimpela, A. and Rantanen, P. (1999) Bullying, depression, and suicidal ideation in Finnish adolescents: school survey. *British Medical Journal 319*, 348–351.

Kandel, D.B., Raveis, V.H. and Davies, M. (1991) Suicidal ideation in adolescence: depression, substance use, and other risk factors. *Journal of Youth and Adolescence 20*, 289–309.

Kann, L., Kinchen, S.A., Williams, B.I., Ross, J.G., Lowry, R., Grunbaum, J.A. and Kolbe, L.J. (2000) Youth risk behaviour surveillance. United States, 1999. *Morbidity and Mortality Weekly Report 49*, 1–96.

Kapur, N., House, A., Creed, F., Feldman, E., Friedman, T. and Guthrie, E. (1998) Management of deliberate self-poisoning in adults in four teaching hospitals: descriptive study. *British Medical Journal 322*, 1203–1207.

Katz, L.Y., Cox, B.J., Gunasekara, S. and Miller, A.L. (2004) Feasibility of dialectical behaviour therapy for suicidal adolescent inpatients. *Journal of the American Academy of Child and Adolescent Psychiatry 43*, 276–282.

Kazdin, A.E., French, N.H., Unis, A.S., Esveldt-Dawson, K. and Sherrick, R.B. (1983) Hopelessness, depression, suicidal intent among psychiatrically disturbed inpatient children. *Journal of Consulting and Clinical Psychology 51*, 504–510.

Kearney, K.A., Hopkins, R.H., Mauss, A.L. and Weisheit, R.A., (1983) Sample bias resulting from a requirement for written parental consent. *Public Opinion Quarterly 47*, 96–102.

Keller, M.B., McCullough, J.P., Klein, D.N., Arnow, B., Dunner, D.L., Gelenberg, A.J., *et al.* (2000) A comparison of nefazodone, the cognitive behavioural analysis system of psychotherapy, and their combination for the treatment of chronic depression. *New England Journal of Medicine 342*, 1462–1470.

Kelly, J.B. (2000) Children's adjustment in conflicted marriage and divorce: a decade review of research. *Journal of the American Academy of Child and Adolescent Psychiatry 39*, 963–973.

Kerfoot, M., Dyer, E., Harrington, V., Woodham, A. and Harrington, R. (1996) Correlates and short-term course of self-poisoning in adolescents. *British Journal of Psychiatry 168*, 38–42.

Kessler, R.C., Borges, G. and Walters, E.E. (1999) Prevalence of and risk factors for lifetime suicide attempts in the national comorbidity survey. *Archives of General Psychiatry 56*, 617–626.

Kienhorst, C.W.M., De Wilde, E.J., Van Den Bout, J., Diekstra, R.F.W. and Wolters, W.H.G. (1990) Characteristics of suicide attempters in a population-based sample of Dutch adolescents. *British Journal of Psychiatry 156*, 243–248.

Kienhorst, I. (1994) Kurt Cobain. *Crisis 15*, 62–63.

King, C.A., Hovey, J.D., Brand, E. and Wilson, R. (1997) Suicidal adolescents after hospitalisation: parent and family impacts on treatment follow-through. *Journal of the American Academy of Child and Adolescent Psychiatry 36*, 85–93.

Kingsbury, S. Hawton, K., Steinhardt, K. and James, A. (1999) Do adolescents who take overdoses have specific psychological characteristics? A comparative study with psychiatric and community controls. *Journal of the American Academy of Child and Adolescent Psychiatry 38*, 1125–1131.

Klerman, G.L. (1988) The current age of youthful melancholia: evidence for increase in depression in adolescents and young adults. *British Journal of Psychiatry 152*, 4–14.

Klingman, A. and Hochdorf, Z. (1993) Coping with distress and self-harm: the impact of a primary prevention program among adolescents. *Journal of Adolescence 16*, 121–140.

Komro, K.A., Perry, C.L., Williams, C.L., Stigler, M.H., Farbaksh, K. and Veblen-Mortenson, S. (2001) How did project Northland reduce alcohol use among young adolescents? Analysis of mediating variables. *Health Education Research 16*, 59–70.

Kramer, T. and Garralda, M.E. (1998) Psychiatric disorders in adolescents in primary care. *British Journal of Psychiatry 173*, 508–513.

Kreitman, N. and Foster, J. (1991) The construction and selection of predictive scales, with special reference to parasuicide. *British Journal of Psychiatry 159*, 185–192.

Kreitman, N. and Schreiber, M. (1979) Parasuicide in young Edinburgh women, 1968–1975. *Psychological Medicine 9*, 469–479.

Kumpulainen, K., Rasanen, E., Henttonen, I., Almqvist, F., Kresanov, K., Linna, S.L., *et al.* (1999) Bullying and psychiatric symptoms among elementary school-age children. *Child Abuse and Neglect 23*, 1253–1262.

Layte, R. and Jenkinson, C. (1997) Social surveys. In C. Jenkinson (ed) *The Assessment and Evaluation of Health and Medical Care.* Buckingham: Open University Press.

Lazarus, R.S. and Folkman, S. (1984) *Stress, Appraisal and Coping.* New York: Springer.

Lee, R.M. (1993) *Doing Research on Sensitive Subjects.* London: Sage Publications.

Lewis, M.W. and Lewis, A.C. (1996) Peer helping programs: helper role, supervisor training and suicidal behaviour. *Journal of Counselling Development 74*, 307–313.

Lewis, S.A., Johnson, J., Cohen, P., Garcia, M. and Velez, C.N. (1988) Attempted suicide in youth: its relationship to school achievement, education goals and socioeconomic status. *Journal of Abnormal Child Psychology 16*, 459–471.

Lewisham, P.M., Rohde, P., Seeley, J.R. and Baldwin, C.L. (2001) Gender differences in suicide attempts from adolescence to young adulthood. *Journal of the American Academy of Child and Adolescent Psychiatry 40*, 427–434.

Linehan, M.M., Armstrong, H.E., Svarez, A., Allmon, D. and Heard, H.L. (1991) Cognitive behavioural treatment of chronically parasuicidal borderline patients. *Archives of General Psychiatry 48*, 1060–1064.

Linehan, M.M., Camper, P., Chiles, J.A., Strohsahl, K. and Shearin, E. (1987) Interpersonal problem solving and parasuicide. *Cognitive Therapy and Research 11*, 1–12.

Littman, S.K. (1983) The role of the press in the control of suicide epidemics. *Proceedings of the International Association for Suicide Prevention and Crisis Intervention.* Paris: Pergamon Press.

MacLeod, A.K., Pankhania, B., Lee, M. and Mitchell, D. (1997) Parasuicide, depression and the anticipation of positive and negative future experiences. *Psychological Medicine 27*, 973–977.

Mann, J.J., Waternaux, C., Haas, G.L. and Malone, K.M. (1999) Toward a clinical model of suicidal behavior in psychiatric patients. *American Journal of Psychiatry 156*, 181–189.

Marcenko, M.O., Fishman, G. and Friedman, J. (1999) Reexamining adolescent suicidal ideation: a developmental perspective applied to a diverse population. *Journal of Youth and Adolescence 28*, 121–138.

March, J., Silva, S., Petrycki, S., Curry, J., Wells, K., Fairbank, J., *et al.* (2004) Fluoxetine, cognitive-behavioral therapy and their combination for adolescents with depression: Treatment for Adolescents with Depression Study (TADS) randomized controlled trial. *Journal of the American Medical Association 292*, 807–820.

Martin, G. (1996) The influence of television suicide in a normal adolescent population. *Archives of Suicide Research 2*, 103–117.

Martin, G., Clarke, M. and Pearce, C. (1993) Adolescent suicide: music preference as an indicator of vulnerability. *Journal of the American Academy of Child and Adolescent Psychiatry 32*, 530–535.

Marttunen, M.J., Aro, H.M. and Lönnqvist, J. (1993) Adolescence and suicide: a review of psychological autopsy studies. *European Child and Adolescent Psychiatry 2*, 10–18.

Mazza, J.J. (2000) The relationship between posttraumatic stress symptomatology and suicidal behavior in school-based adolescents. *Suicide and Life-Threatening Behavior 30*, 91–103.

McGee, R. and Williams, S. (2000) Does low self-esteem predict health compromising behaviours among adolescents? *Journal of Adolescence 23*, 569–582.

McKenna K.Y.A. and Bargh, J. (1998) Coming out in the age of the Internet. Identity demarginalization through virtual group participation. *Journal of Personality and Social Psychology 75*, 681–694.

MediaWise Trust (2003) Suicide and the Media. http://presswise.org.uk/display_page.php?id =166. Accessed 9 August 2005.

Meltzer, H., Harrington, R., Goodman, R. and Jenkins, R. (2001) *Children and Adolescents Who Try to Harm, Hurt or Kill Themselves.* London: Office for National Statistics.

Merrill, J. and Owens, J. (1986) Ethnic differences in self-poisoning: a comparison of Asian and white groups. *British Journal of Psychiatry 148*, 708–712.

Michaud, P.A. and Fombonne, E. (2005) Common mental health problems. *British Medical Journal 330*, 835–838.

Michel, K. (2000) Suicide prevention and primary care. In K. Hawton and K. Van Heeringen (eds) *The International Handbook of Suicide and Attempted Suicide.* Chichester: John Wiley & Sons.

Michel, K. Frey, C., Wyss, K. and Valach, L. (2000) An exercise in improving suicide reporting in print media. *Crisis 21*, 1–10.

Michel, K., Runeson, B., Valach, L. and Wasserman, D. (1997) Contacts of suicide attempters with GPs prior to the event: a comparison between Stockholm and Bern. *Acta Psychiatrica Scandinavica 95*, 94–99.

Midanik, L.T. (1988) Validity of self-reported alcohol use: a literature review and assessment. *British Journal of Addiction 83*, 1019–1030.

Miller, D.N. and DuPaul, G.J. (1996) School-based prevention of adolescent suicide: issues, obstacles and recommendations for practice. *Journal of Emotional and Behavioural Disorders 4*, 221–230.

Mills, J., Williams, C., Sale, I., Perkin, G. and Henderson, S. (1974) The epidemiology of self-poisoning in Hobart, 1968–1972. *Australian and New Zealand Journal of Psychiatry 8*, 167–172.

Monck, E., Graham, P., Richman, N. and Dobbs, R. (1994) Adolescent girls. I: selfreported mood disturbance in a community population. *British Journal of Psychiatry 165*, 760–769.

Morgan, H.G., Jones, E.M. and Owen, J.H. (1993) Secondary prevention of non-fatal attempted suicide. *British Journal of Psychiatry 163*, 111–112.

Murray, D.M. and Fisher, J.D. (2002) The Internet: a virtually untapped tool for research. *Journal of Technology in Human Sciences 19*, 5–18.

National Institute for Clinical Excellence (2004) *Clinical Guideline 16. Self-harm: The Short-term Physical and Psychological Management and Secondary Prevention of Self-harm in Primary and Secondary Care.* London: National Institute for Clinical Excellence.

National Institute for Clinical Excellence (2005) *Depression in Children and Young People: Identification and Management in Primary, Community and Secondary Care.* London: National Institute for Clinical Excellence.

National Suicide Research Foundation (2004) *National Parasuicide Registry Ireland: Annual Report 2003*. Cork: National Suicide Research Foundation.

Neeleman, J. and Wessely, S. (1999) Ethnic minority suicide: a small area geographical study in South London. *Psychological Medicine 29*, 429–436.

Nicholas, J., Oliver, K., Lee, K. and O'Brien, M. (2004) Help-seeking and the Internet: an investigation among Australian adolescents. *Australian e-Journal for the Advancement of Mental Health 3*. Accessible at www.ausienet.com/journal/vol3iss1/nicholas.pdf.

Nosek, B.A., Banaji, M.R. and Greenwald, A.G. (2002) e-Research: ethics, security, design and control in psychological research on the Internet. *Journal of Social Issues 58*, 161–176.

O'Grady, J. (1999) Acute liver failure. *Medicine 27*, 80–82.

Oliver, R.G., Kaminski, Z., Tudor, K. and Hertzel, B.S. (1971) The epidemiology of attempted suicide as seen in the casualty department, Alfred Hospital, Melbourne. *Medical Journal of Australia 1*, 833–839.

O'Loughlin, S. and Sherwood, J. (2005) A 20-year review of trends in deliberate self-harm in a British town, 1981–2000. *Social Psychiatry and Psychiatric Epidemiology 40*, 446–453.

Olsson, G. and Von Knorring, A.L. (1999) Adolescent depression: prevalence in Swedish high school students. *Acta Psychiatrica Scandinavica 99*, 324–331.

Otto, U. (1972) Suicidal acts by children and adolescents: a follow-up study. *Acta Psychiatrica Scandinavica Supplementum 233*, 96.

Overholser, J.C., Adams, D.M., Lehnert, K.L. and Brinkman, D.C. (1995) Self-esteem deficits and suicidal tendencies among adolescents. *Journal of the American Academy of Child and Adolescent Psychiatry 34, 919–928*.

Overholser, J.C., Huston Hemstreet, A., Spirito, A. and Vyse, S. (1989) Suicide awareness programs in schools: effects of gender and personal experience. *Journal of American Academy of Child and Adolescent Psychiatry 28*, 925–930.

Owens, D., Horrocks, J. and House, A. (2002) Fatal and non-fatal repetition of self-harm. *British Journal of Psychiatry 181*, 193–199.

Oxfordshire Adolescent Self-Harm Forum (2004) *Self-harm: Guidelines for School Staff*, 2nd edn. Oxford: Oxfordshire Adolescent Self-Harm Forum.

Pagès, F., Arvers, P., Hassler, C. and Choquet, M. (2004) What are the characteristics of adolescent hospitlaised suicide attempters? *European Child and Adolescent Psychiatry 13*, 151–158.

Patton, G.C., Harris, R., Carlin, J.B., Hibbert, M.E., Coffey, C., Schwarz, M. and Bowes, G. (1997) Adolescent suicidal behaviours: a population based study of risk. *Psychological Medicine 27*, 715–724.

Patton, G.C., Glover, S., Bond, L., Butler, H., Godfrey, C., Di-Petro, G. and Bowes, G. (2000) The Gatehouse Projects: a systematic approach to mental health promotion in secondary schools. *Australian and New Zealand Journal of Psychiatry 34*, 586–593.

Pearce, C.M. and Martin, G. (1993) Locus of control as an indicator of risk for suicidal behaviour among adolescents. *Acta Psychiatrica Scandinavica 88*, 409–414.

Pfeffer, C.R., McBride, A., Anderson, G.M., Kakuma, T., Fensterheim, L. and Khait, V. (1998) Peripheral serotonin measures in pre-pubertal psychiatric inpatients and normal children: associations with suicidal behaviour and its risk factors. *Biological Psychiatry 44*, 569–577.

Phillips, D.P. (1974) The influence of suggestion on suicide: substantive and theoretical implications of the Werther effect. *American Sociological Review 39*, 340–354.

Phillips, D.P. (1980) Airplane accidents, murder and the mass media: towards a theory of imitation and suggestion. *Social Forces 58*, 1001–1024.

Pilowsky, D.J., Wu, L. and Anthony, J.C. (1999) Panic attacks and suicide attempts in mid-adolescence. *American Journal of Psychiatry 156*, 1545–1549.

Pirkis, J. and Blood, R.W. (2001) *Suicide and the Media: A Critical Review.* Canberra: Commonwealth Department of Health and Aged Care.

Platt, S., Bille-Brahe, U., Kerkhof, A., Schmidtke, A., Bjerke, T., Crepet, P., *et al.* (1992) Parasuicide in Europe: the WHO/EURO multicentre study on parasuicide. Introduction and preliminary analysis for 1989. *Acta Psychiatrica Scandinavica 85*, 97–104.

Platt, S., Hawton, K., Kreitman, N., Fagg, J. and Foster, J. (1988) Recent clinical and epidemiological trends in parasuicide in Edinburgh and Oxford: a tale of two cities. *Psychological Medicine 18*, 405–418.

Plutchik, R. and Van Praag, H.M. (1986) The measurement of suicidality, aggressivity and impulsivity. *Clinical Neuropharmacology 9*, 380–382.

Poijula, S., Wahlberg, K.E. and Dyregrov, A. (2001) Adolescent suicide and suicide contagion in three secondary schools. *International Journal of Emergency Mental Health 3*, 163–168.

Poland, S. (1995) Suicide intervention. In A. Thomas and J. Grimes (eds) *Best Practices in School Psychology III.* Washington, DC: National Association of School Psychologists.

Ponizovsky, A.M., Ritsner, M.S. and Modai, I. (1999) Suicidal ideation and suicide attempts among immigrant adolescents from the former Soviet Union to Israel. *Journal of the American Academy of Child and Adolescent Psychiatry 38*, 1433–1441.

Qin, P. and Mortensen, P.B. (2003) The impact of parental stress on the risk of completed suicide. *Archives of General Psychiatry 60*, 797–802.

Rahman, A., Mubbashar, M.H., Gater, R. and Goldberg, D. (1998) Randomised trial of impact of a school mental-health programme in rural Rawalpindi, Pakistan. *Lancet 352*, 1022–1025.

Raleigh, S. and Balarajan, R. (1992) Suicide and self-burning among Indians and West Indians in England and Wales. *British Journal of Psychiatry 161*, 365–368.

Raviv, A., Sills, R., Raviv, A. and Wilansky, P. (2000) Adolescents' help-seeking behaviour: the difference between self- and other referral. *Journal of Adolescence 23*, 721–70.

Reinherz, H.Z., Giaconia, R.M., Silverman, A.B., *et al.* (1995) Early psychosocial risks for adolescent suicidal ideation and attempts. *Journal of American Academy of Child and Adolescent Psychiatry 34*, 599–611.

Reith, D., Whyte, I. and Carter, G. (2003) Repetition of risk for adolescent self-poisoning: a multiple event survival analysis. *Australian and New Zealand Journal of Psychiatry 37*, 212–218.

Rey Gex, C.R., Narring, F., Ferron, C. and Michaud, P.A. (1998) Suicide attempts among adolescents in Switzerland: prevalence, associated factors and comorbidity. *Acta Psychiatrica Scandinavica 98*, 28–33.

Reynolds, W.M. (1987) *Adult Suicidal Ideation Questionnaire.* Odessa, FL: Psychological Assessment Resources.

Reynolds, W.M. (1990) Development of a semi-structured clinical interview for suicidal behaviours in adolescents. *Psychological Assessment 2*, 382–390.

Reynolds, W.M. (1991) A school-based procedure for the identification of adolescents at risk for suicidal behaviours. *Family and Community Health 14*, 64–75.

Reynolds, W.M. and Mazza, J.J. (1994) Suicide and suicidal behaviours in children and adolescents. In W.M. Reynolds and H.F. Johnston (eds) *Handbook of Depression in Children and Adolescents.* New York: Plenum Press.

Rigby, K. and Slee, P. (1999) Suicidal ideation among adolescent school children, involvement in bully-victim problems and perceived social support. *Suicide and Life-Threatening Behavior 29,* 119–130.

Roberts, R.E., Chen, Y.R. and Roberts, C.R. (1997) Ethnocultural differences in prevalence of adolescent suicidal behaviors. *Suicide and Life-Threatening Behavior 27,* 208–217.

Robson, P. (1989) Development of a new self-report questionnaire to measure self-esteem. *Psychological Medicine 19,* 513–518.

Rodham, K., Hawton, K. and Evans, E. (2004) Reasons for deliberate self-harm: comparison of self-poisoners and self-cutters in a community sample of adolescents. *Journal of the American Academy of Child and Adolescent Psychiatry 43,* 80–87.

Rossow, I. and Wichstrøm, L. (1994) Parasuicide and use of intoxicants among Norwegian adolescents. *Suicide and Life-Threatening Behavior 24,* 174–183.

Rotheram-Borus, M.J., Trautman, P.D., Dopkins, S.C. and Shrout, P.E. (1990) Cognitive style and pleasant activities among female adolescent suicide attempters. *Journal of Consulting and Clinical Psychology 58,* 554–561.

Roy, A. (2000) Relation of family history of suicide to suicide attempts in alcoholics. *American Journal of Psychiatry 157,* 2050–2051.

Royal College of General Practitioners and Royal College of Nursing (2002) *Getting it Right for Teenagers in Your Practice.* London: Royal College of General Practitioners and Royal College of Nursing.

Royal College of Paediatrics and Child Health (2003) *Bridging the Gaps: Healthcare for Adolescents.* London: Royal College of Paediatrics and Child Health.

Royal College of Psychiatrists (1994) *The general hospital management of adult deliberate self-harm.* Council report CR32. London: Royal College of Psychiatrists.

Royal College of Psychiatrists (1998) *Managing Deliberate Self-harm in Young People.* Council Report R64. London: Royal College of Psychiatrists.

Royal College of Psychiatrists (2004) *Assessment Following Self-harm in Adults.* London: Royal College of Psychiatrists.

Rubenstein, J.L., Heeren, T., Housman, D., Rubin, C. and Stechler, G. (1989) Suicidal behavior in 'normal' adolescents: risk and protective factors. *American Journal of Orthopsychiatry 59,* 59–71.

Runeson, B.S, Beskow, J. and Waern, M. (1996) The suicidal process in suicides among young people. *Acta Psychiatrica Scandinavica 93,* 35–42.

Rustard, R.A., Small, J.E., Jobes, D.A., Safer, M.A. and Peterson, R.J. (2003) The impact of rock viedoes and music with suicidal content on thoughts and attitudes about suicide. *Suicide and Life-Threateneing Behavior, 33,* 120–131.

Rutter, M., Taylor, E. and Hersov, M. (1994) *Child and Adolescent Psychiatry: Modern Approaches,* 3rd edn. Oxford: Blackwell Science.

Sacco, W.P. and Graves, D.J. (1984) Childhood depression, interpersonal problemsolving and self-ratings of performance. *Journal of Clinical Child Psychology 13,* 10–15.

Sadowski, C., and Kelly, M. (1993) Social problem-solving in suicidal adolescents. *Journal of Consulting and Clinical Psychology 61,* 121–127.

Safer, D. (1997a) Adolescent/adult differences in suicidal behaviour and outcome. *Annals of Clinical Psychiatry 9,* 61–66.

Safer, D. J. (1997b) Self-reported suicide attempts by adolescents. *Annals of Clinical Psychiatry 9,* 263–269.

Sakinofsky, I. (2000) Repetition of suicidal behaviour. In K. Hawton, and K. Van Heeringen (eds) *The International Handbook of Suicide and Attempted Suicide.* Chichester: John Wiley & Sons.

Salmons, P.H. and Harrington, R. (1984) Suicidal ideation in university students and other groups. *International Journal of Social Psychiatry 30*, 201–205.

Samaritans (2002) *Media Guidelines: Portrayal of Suicide.* Ewell: Samaritans.

Sanci, L.A., Coffey, C.M., Veit, F.C., Carr-Gregg, M., Patton, G.C., Day, N. and Bowes, G. (2000) Evaluation of the effectiveness of an educational intervention for general practitioners in adolescent health care: randomised controlled trial. *British Medical Journal 320*, 224–230.

Sargent, J.D., Dalton, M.A., Beach, M.L., Mott, L.A., Tickle, J.J., Ahrens, M.B. and Heatherton, T.F. (2002) Viewing tobacco use in movies: does it shape attitudes that mediate adolescent smoking? *American Journal of Preventive Medicine 22*, 137–145.

Saunders, S.M., Resnick, M.D., Hoberman, H.M. and Blum, R.W. (1994) Formal help-seeking behaviour of adolescents identifying themselves as having mental health problems. *Journal of the American Academy of Child and Adolescent Psychiatry 33*, 718–728.

Scheel, K.R. and Westfield, J.S. (1999) Heavy metal music and adolescent suicidality: an empirical investigation. *Adolescence 34*, 253–273.

Schmidt, U. and Davidson, K. (2004) *Life After Self-harm: A Guide to the Future.* Hove: Brunner-Routledge.

Schmidtke, A. and Häfner, H. (1988) The Werther effect after television films: new evidence for an old hypothesis. *Psychological Medicine 18*, 665–676.

Schmidtke, A. and Schaller, S. (2000) The role of mass media in suicide prevention. In K. Hawton and K. Van Heeringeen (eds) *The International Handbook of Suicide and Attempted Suicide.* Chichester: John Wiley & Sons.

Schmidtke, A., Bille-Brahe, U., De Leo, D., Kerkhof, A., Bjerke, T., Crepet, P., *et al.* (1996) Attempted suicide in Europe: rates, trends and sociodemographic characteristics of suicide attempters during the period 1989–1992. Results of the WHO/EURO Multicentre Study on Parasuicide. *Acta Psychiatrica Scandinavica 93*, 327–338.

Schonert-Reichl, K.A. and Muller, J.R. (1996) Correlates of help-seeking in adolescence. *Journal of Youth and Adolescence 25*, 705–731.

Schotte, D.E. and Clum, G.A. (1987) Problem-solving skills in suicidal psychiatric patients. *Journal of Consulting and Clinical Psychology 55*, 49–54.

Sell, L. and Robson, P. (1998) Perceptions of college life, emotional well-being and patterns of drug and alcohol use among Oxford undergraduates. *Oxford Review of Education 24*, 235–243.

Sellar, C., Hawton, K. and Goldacre, M. (1990) Self-poisoning in adolescents: hospital admissions and deaths in the Oxford region. *British Journal of Psychiatry 156*, 866–870.

Shaffer, D. and Craft, L. (1999) Methods of adolescent suicide prevention. *Journal of Clinical Psychiatry 60*, 70–74.

Shaffer, D., Garland, A., Gould, M., Fisher, P. and Trautman, P. (1988) Preventing teenage suicide: a critical review. *Journal of the American Academy of Child and Adolescent Psychiatry 27*, 675–687.

Shaffer, D., Garland, A., Vieland, V., Underwood, M.M. and Busner, C. (1991) The impact of a curriculum-based suicide prevention program for teenagers. *Journal of the American Academy of Child and Adolescent Psychiatry 30*, 588–596.

Shaffer, D. and Gould, M. (2000) Suicide prevention in schools. In K. Hawton and K. Van Heeringen (eds) *The International Handbook of Suicide and Attempted Suicide.* Chichester: John Wiley & Sons.

Shaffer, D., Gould, M., Fisher, P., Trautman, P., Moreau, D., Kleinman, M. and Flory, M. (1996) Psychiatric diagnosis in child and adolescent suicide. *Archives of General Psychiatry 53*, 339–348.

Shaffer, D, Scott, M., Wilcox, Hl, Maslwo, C., Hicks, R., Lucas, C.P., *et al* (2004) The Columbia Suicide Screen: validity and reliability of a screen for youth suicide and depression. *Journal of the American Academy of Child and Adolescent Psychiatry 43,* 71–79.

Shaffer, D., Vieland, V., Garland, A., Rojas, M., Underwood, M. and Busner, C. (1990) Adolescent suicide attempters: response to suicide-prevention programs. *Journal of American Medical Association 264*, 3151–3155.

Shafi, M., Carrigan, S., Whittinghill, J.R. and Derrick, A. (1985) Psychological autopsy of completed suicide in children and adolescents. *American Journal of Psychiatry 142*, 1061–1064.

Sharp, D.J., Liebanau, A.I., Stocks, N., Evans, M., Bruce-Jones, W., Peters, T.J., *et al.* (2003) Locally developed guidelines for the aftercare of deliberate self-harm patients in general practice. *Primary Health Care 4*, 21–28.

Shearer, S.L. (1994) Phenomenology of self-injury among inpatient women with borderline personality disorder. *Journal of Nervous and Mental Disease 182*, 524–526.

Shochet, I.M. and O'Gorman, J.G. (1995) Ethical issues in research on adolescent depression and suicidal behaviour. *Australian Psychologist 30*, 183–186.

Silbert, K.L. and Berry, G.L. (1991) Psychological effects of a suicide prevention unit on adolescents' levels of stress, anxiety and hopelessness: implications for counselling psychologists. *Counselling Psychologist 4*, 45–58.

Simons, R.L. and Murphy, P.I. (1985) Sex differences in the causes of adolescent suicide ideation. *Journal of Youth and Adolescence 14*, 423–434.

Smart D., Pollard, C. and Walpole, B. (1999) Mental health triage in emergency medicine. *Australian and New Zealand Journal of Psychiatry 33*, 57–66.

Sonneck, G., Etzerdorfer, E. and Nagel-Kuess, S. (1994) Imitative suicide on the Viennese subway. *Social Science and Medicine 38*, 453–457.

Speckens, A.E.M. and Hawton, K. (2005) Social problem-solving in adolescents with suicidal behaviour: a systematic review. *Suicide and Life-Threatening Behavior 35*, 365–457.

Stack, S. (1991) Social correlates of suicide by age: media impacts. In A. Leenaars (ed) *Life-span Perspectives of Suicide Time-lines in the Suicide Process.* New York: Plenum Press.

Stanley, E.J. and Barter, J.T. (1970) Adolescent suicidal behaviour. *American Journal of Orthopsychiatry 40*, 87.

Statham, D., Heath, A., Madden, P., Bucholz, K., Dinwiddie, S., Slutake, W., *et al.* (1998) Suicidal behaviour: an epidemiological and genetic study. *Psychological Medicine 28*, 839–855.

Stewart, S.M., Lam, T.H., Betson, C. and Chung, S.F. (1999) Suicide ideation and its relationship to depressed mood in a community sample of adolescents in Hong Kong. *Suicide and Life-Threatening Behavior 29*, 227–240.

Stork, V.J. (1972) Suizidtendenz und suizidversuch statistische analyse des suizidalen feldes bei schülern. *Zeitschrift fur Klinische Psychologie und Psychotherapie 20*, 123–151.

Straus, M.A. and Kantor, G.K. (1994) Corporal punishment of adolescents by parents: a risk factor in the epidemiology of depression, suicide, alcohol abuse, child abuse, and wife beating. *Adolescence 29*, 543–561.

Sullivan, C., Corcoran, P., Arensman, E. and Perry, I.J. (submitted) The prevalence of self-reported deliberate self-harm in Irish adolescents.

Swanson, J.W., Linskey, A.O., Quintero, S.R., Pumariega, A.J. and Holzer, C.E. (1992) A bi-national school survey of depressive symptoms, drug use and suicidal ideation. *Journal of the American Academy of Child and Adolescent Psychiatry 31*, 669–678.

Takahashi, Y. (1998) Suicide in Japan. What are the problems? In R.J. Kosky, H.S. Eshkevari, R.D. Goldney and R. Hassan (eds) *Suicide Prevention*. New York: Plenum Press.

Taylor, E.A. and Stansfeld, S.A. (1984a) Children who poison themselves: I. A clinical comparison with psychiatric controls. *British Journal of Psychiatry 145*, 127–132.

Taylor, E.A. and Stansfeld, S.A. (1984b) Children who poison themselves: II. Prediction of attendance for treatment. *British Journal of Psychiatry 145*, 132–135.

Thompson, K.M., Wonderlich, S.A., Crosby, R.D. and Mitchell, J.E. (1999) The neglected link between eating disturbances and aggressive behaviour in girls. *Journal of the American Academy of Child and Adolescent Psychiatry 38*, 1277–1284.

Tomori, M. (1999) Suicide risk in high school students in Slovenia. *Crisis 20*, 23–27.

Tomori, M. and Rus-Makovec, M. (2000) Eating behaviour, depression and self-esteem in high school students. *Journal of Adolescent Health 26*, 361–367.

Townsend, E., Hawton, K., Altman, D.G., Arensman, E., Gunnell, D., Hazell, P., *et al.* (2001) The efficacy of problem-solving treatments after deliberate self-harm: meta-analysis of randomised controlled trails with respect to depression, hopelessness and improvement in problems. *Psychological Medicine 31*, 979–988.

Underwood, M.M. and Dunne-Maxim, K. (1997) *Managing sudden traumatic loss in Schools*. Newark, NJ: University of Medicine and Dentistry of New Jersey.

UK Medicine and Healthcare Products Regulatory Agency: Committee on Safety of Medicines (2004) www.medicines.mhra.gov.uk. Accessed 24 August 2005.

US Food and Drug Administration (2004). US Food and Drug Administration: www.fda.gov/cder /drug/antidepressants/AntidepressantsPHA.htm. Accessed 24 August 2005.

Vajda, J. and Steinbeck, K. (2000) Factors associated with repeat suicide attempts among adolescents. *Australian and New Zealand Journal of Psychiatry 34*, 437–445.

Van Casteren, V., Van der Veken, J., Tafforeau, J. and Van Oyen, H. (1993) Suicide and attempted suicide reported by general practitioners in Belgium. *Acta Psychiatrica Scandinavica 87*, 451–455.

Van Heeringen, C. (2000) Suicide in adolescents. *European Psychiatry 15*, 248S.

Van Heeringen, C. and De Volder, V. (2002) Trends in attempted suicide in adolescents and young adults, 1986–1995. *Archives of Suicide Research 6*, 135–143.

Van Heeringen, C. and Vincke, J. (2000) Suicidal acts and ideation in homosexual and bisexual young people: a study of prevalence and risk factors. *Social Psychiatry and Psychiatric Epidemiology 35*, 494–499.

Van Heeringen, K. (2001) *Understanding Suicidal Behavioour: The Suicidal Process Approach to Research, Treatment and Prevention*. Chichester: John Wiley & Sons.

Vannatta, R.A. (1996) Risk factors related to suicidal behavior among male and female adolescents. *Journal of Youth and Adolescence 25*, 149–160.

Vignau, J., Bailly, D., Duhamel, A., Vervaecke, P., Beuscart, R. and Collinet, C. (1997) Epidemiologic study of sleep quality and troubles in French secondary school adolescents. *Journal of Adolescent Health 21*, 343–350.

Viner, R. and MacFarlane, A. (2005) Health promotion. *British Medical Journal 330*, 527–529.

Volkmar, F.R. (1996) Childhood and adolescent psychosis: a review of the past 10 years. *Journal of the American Academy of Child and Adolescent Psychiatry 35*, 843–851.

Wagman Borowsky, I., Resnick, M.D., Ireland, M. and Blum, R.W. (1999) Suicide attempts among American Indian and Alaska native youth. *Archives of Pediatric and Adolescent Medicine 153*, 573–580.

Wagner, B.M., Cole, R.E. and Schwartzman, P. (1995) Psychosocial correlates of suicide attempts among junior and senior high school youth. *Suicide and Life-Threatening Behavior 25*, 358–372.

Wagner, B.M., Aiken, C., Mullaley, P.M. and Tobin, J.J. (2000) Parents' reactions to adolescents' suicide attempts. *Journal of the American Academy of Child and Adolescent Psychiatry 39*, 429–436.

Wainwright, D. and Calnan, M. (2002) *Work Stress: The Making of a Modern Epidemic*. Buckingham: Open University Press.

Wallace, P. (1999) *The Psychology of the Internet*. Cambridge: Cambridge University Press.

Walsh, B.W. and Rosen, P.M. (1989) *Self-mutilation: Theory, Research and Treatment*. New York: The Guilford Press.

Walter, H.J., Vaughan, R.D., Armstrong, B., Krakoff, R.Y., Tiezzi, L. and McCarthy, J.F. (1995) Characteristics of users and nonusers of health clinics in inner-city junior high schools. *Journal of Adolescent Health 18*, 348.

Walther, J.B. and Boyd, S. (2002) Attraction to computer-mediated social support. In C.A. Lin and D. Atkin (eds) *Communication Technology and Society: Audience Adoption and Uses*. Cresskill, NJ: Hampton Press.

Wellman, B. (1997) An electronic group is virtually a social network. In S. Kiesler (ed) *Culture of the Internet*. Mahwah, NJ: Lawrence Erlbaum.

Wells, J., Barlow, J. and Stewart-Brown, S. (2003) A systematic review of universal approaches to mental health promotion in schools. *Health Education 103*, 197–220.

West, P. and Sweeting, H. (2003) 'Fifteen, female and stressed: changing patterns of psychological distress over time'. *Journal of Child Psychology and Psychiatry 44*, 399–411.

Wexler, L., Weissman, M.M. and Kasl, S.V. (1978) Suicide attempts 1970–75: updating a United States study and comparisons with international trends. *Archives of General Psychiatry 132*, 180–185.

White, D., Leach, C., Sims, R., Atkinson, M. and Cottrell, D. (1999) Validation of the Hospital Anxiety and Depression Scale for use with adolescents. *British Journal of Psychiatry 175*, 452–454.

Whittington, C.J., Kendall, T., Fonagy, P., Cottrell, D., Cotgrove, A. and Boddington, E. (2004) Selective serotonin reuptake inhibitors in childhood depression: systematic review of published versus unpublished data. *Lancet 363*, 1341–1345.

Williams, J.M.G. (1997) *Cry of Pain: Understanding Suicide and Self-harm*. Harmondsworth: Penguin.

Williams, J.M.G. and Pollock, L.R. (2000) The psychology of suicidal behaviour. In K. Hawton and K. van Heeringen (eds) *The International Handbook of Suicide and Attempted Suicide*. Chichester: John Wiley & Sons.

Wilson, H.W. (2003) Staff knowledge and attitudes towards deliberate self-harm in adolescents. *Journal of Adolescence 26*, 623.

Wood, A., Trainor, G., Rothwell, J., Moore, A. and Harrington, R. (2001) Randomized trial of group therapy for repeated deliberate self-harm in adolescents. *Journal of the American Academy of Child and Adolescent Psychiatry 40*, 1246–1253.

World Health Organization (1993) *The ICD-10 Classification of Mental and Behavioural Disorders: Diagnostic Criteria for Research*. Geneva: World Health Organization.

Wright, K.B. (2000) Perceptions of on-line support providers: an examination of perceived homophily, source credibility, communication and social support within online support groups. *Communication Quarterly 48*, 44–59.

Wright, K.B. and Bell, S.B. (2003) Health-related support groups on the Internet: linking empirical findings to social support and computer-mediated communication theory. *Journal of Health Psychology 8*, 39–54.

Wright, L.S. (1985) Suicidal thoughts and their relationship to family stress and personal problems among high school seniors and college undergraduates. *Adolescence 20*, 575–580.

Wyn, J., Cahill, H., Holdsworth, R., Rowling, L. and Carson, S. (2000) Mindmatters: a whole-school approach promoting mental health and wellbeing. *Australian and New Zealand Journal of Psychiatry 34*, 594–601.

Ystgaard, M., Reinholdt, N.P., Husby, J. and Mehlum, L. (2003) [Deliberate self-harm in adolescents.] *Tidisskrift for den Norske laegeforening 123*, 2241–2245.

Yuen, N., Andrade, N., Nahulu, L., Makini, G., McDermott, J.F., Danko, G., *et al.* (1996) The rate and characteristics of suicide attempters in the native Hawaiian adolescent population. *Suicide and Life-Threatening Behavior 26*, 27–36.

Zahl, D. and Hawton, K. (2004) Repetition of deliberate self-harm and subsequent suicide risk: long term follow-up study in 11,583 patients. *British Journal of Psychiatry 185*, 70–75.

Zigmond, A.S. and Snaith, R.P. (1983) The Hospital Anxiety and Depression Scale. *Acta Psychiatrica Scandinavica 67*, 361–370.

Subject Index

Author Index